THE NURSE'S COMMUNICATION HANDBOOK

Harry E. Munn, Jr., Ph.D.

Associate Professor
North Carolina State University
Raleigh, North Carolina

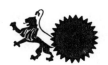

AN ASPEN PUBLICATION®
Aspen Systems Corporation
Germantown, Maryland
London, England
1980

Library of Congress Cataloging in Publication Data

Munn, Harry E.
The nurse's communication handbook.

Includes bibliographies and index.

1. Communication in nursing.   I. Title. [DNLM:
1. Communication—Nursing texts.   2. Communication—
Handbooks.   3. Nurse-patient relations—Handbooks.
WY87 M966n]
RT23.M86   610.73   80-13066
ISBN: 0-89443-284-2

Library of Congress Catalog Card Number: 80-13066
ISBN: 0-89443-284-2

Printed in the United States of America

1 2 3 4 5

To My Father,

who, over the years, has been interested in and contributed to the work of the Shriners' hospitals for crippled children. He has played an integral part in my life, in the lives of others, and can never be repaid for what he has done.

And to the Shriners,

the many thousands of them, who have given of themselves for such noble work.

Table of Contents

Preface

Communication is as necessary to an organization as the bloodstream is to a person. Just as the bloodstream must flow unhindered, communication must flow freely. The bloodstream must be responsive to the internal needs of the body. Likewise, communication must be responsive to the internal needs of the organization. This communicative responsiveness requires one to develop an ability to communicate clearly, concisely, and with understanding.

Based on these precepts, this nursing handbook is intended for use by schools of nursing, health care facilities, and hospital training programs. It is meant to be practical and concise and was written for the following reasons:

1. Nurses are constantly exchanging information via communication, but they may have only limited knowledge of interpersonal or small group communication processes.

2. The communicative behavior of nurses with and among other health care professionals and patients will ultimately affect the mental and physical well-being of their patients.

3. Nurses can improve their communicative knowledge and behavior only through instruction in interpersonal and small group processes.

4. Nurses have a professional need to be able to diagnose communicative illness and then be able to employ appropriate treatment.

5. Nurses must be able to apply this treatment, if necessary, in a health care setting.

6. Nurses might have an abundant supply of medical knowledge,

but communication is the only tool they have with which to exchange this knowledge with others. To be able to share and understand information is the only way an individual or organization can maintain excellent communicative health.

Acknowledgments

This book would not have been possible without the help of Gordon Marshall, editor and publisher of *Hospital Topics,* and Marcella Marshall, assistant to the publisher. Both provided this writer with encouragement and the opportunity to share experiences with other health care professionals.

Grateful acknowledgment is also extended to the nurses and other health care professionals who provided many of the examples used in this book. Special appreciation is reserved for Jo Anne Brooks, Southeastern Medical Records Association; Boyd Gillis, North Carolina Division of Mental Health; Commander Shirley Hicks, Portsmouth Naval Regional Medical Center; Dr. Rebecca Leonard, North Carolina State University; Ruth Martin, Associate Director of Nursing, District of Columbia General Hospital; Robert McLain, North Carolina Hospital Personnel Association; Thelma Parsons, Director of In-Service Education, Wake County Hospital Systems; Alvin Resnick, Vice-President, Unicare Health Facilities; Wayne Smith, John Umstead Hospital; and Joan Spear, Baltimore Chapter, Association of Operating Room Nurses.

Final appreciation goes to two special friends: Dr. Bill Conboy, University of Kansas, who provided many of the original ideas for this book, and Dr. Bill Franklin, Chairman of the Department of Speech Communication, North Carolina State University, who provided the original impetus for the book through encouragement, understanding, and guidance.

Chapter 1

Motivation for Nurses through Nurses

CHAPTER OBJECTIVES

The purpose of this chapter is to enable you to
CHANGE your communicative behavior in a
positive direction. After studying the material
you should be able to:

Compare your motivational needs to those of
other nurses.

Have an understanding of various motivational
theories.

Assess your personal motivational needs and
be able to rank order them in respect to their
importance to *you.*

Name and employ motivational theories that
are applicable to your job.

Guide yourself and your peers to meet the
motivational needs of others.

Encourage *positive* thinking within your work
group.

T he nurse invariably joins the profession for one reason: to help people. Nurses, in the truest sense of the word, are in the people business; but amid bedpans, thermometers, government regulations, meetings, and medical charts the nurse's enthusiasm tends to wane. The National League for Nursing (NLN) reports (1979) that only 69.7 percent of the nation's nurses remain in the field ten years after graduation. Some sources say that figure is too high and estimate that most nurses stay in the field from one and one-half to three years.

In school nurses are taught to care for the patients' emotional and physical needs, but little time is spent discussing how nurses can meet their own emotional and physical needs within the hospital setting. Many nurses report they have no time for hobbies, are emotionally drained when they go home, and have no time for anything but nursing. They eat, sleep, and think nursing.

This country prides itself on the quality of health care available to its citizens. However, this concern for quality care can be quickly eroded if we neglect the care of the people performing that service. Hospitals today are a big business; and, like any successful business, they must meet the needs of their employees.

EMPLOYEE NEEDS

Nurses, nursing supervisors, and hospital administrators at the seventh annual *Hospital Topics* Nursing Convention, held in 1979 in Chicago, were asked to rank the following items. They ranked the items first with respect to their importance to them personally and then with respect to how they thought their employees would rank them. How do you rank these items in terms of their importance to you? Each item is to be given one numerical value, one denoting the most important and ten the least important.

The Needs of the Health Care Professional

Your Rating		Nurses' Rating	Supervisors' Rating
_____	Appreciation of Work Done.	_____	_____
_____	Feeling "in" on Things.	_____	_____
_____	Professional Growth.	_____	_____
_____	Challenging Work.	_____	_____
_____	Good Wages.	_____	_____
_____	Good Working Conditions.	_____	_____
_____	Management Loyalty to Workers.	_____	_____
_____	Promotion.	_____	_____
_____	Help on Personal Problems.	_____	_____
_____	Tactful Disciplining.	_____	_____

You might also want to make an educated guess as to how the nurses, nursing supervisors, and hospital administrators responded to the items. The results of the survey are presented later in this chapter.

MOTIVATIONAL THEORY

Douglas McGregor has noted that theory is a most practical matter. Without underlying beliefs and assumptions we would be unable to act aside from our reflexive responses. Theory and practice are inseparable.[1]

Every time a nurse administers care to a patient, there is a theoretic premise behind that action. Therefore, an understanding of motivational theory can enable the nurse to respond in a reflective rather than a reflexive manner.

The early work of Abraham Maslow still serves as the main source of motivational theory today. Maslow contended that we are motivated by a hierarchy of human needs. This hierarchy takes the shape of a ladder. The first rung represents our basic need for food, clothing and shelter. When this need is satisfied, we climb to the second rung: our need to feel safe from harm or injury. We then climb to the third rung: our need to associate with family and friends. The fourth rung represents our esteem needs, to be well liked and respected. Finally, the top rung represents self-actualization needs, the need to grow and become whatever we are capable of becoming.[2]

On this ladder of human needs, we can see that we hop up and down the rungs every day of our lives. The survey you responded to earlier touches upon each of these human needs.

SELF–ACTUALIZATION
_____

ESTEEM
_____

BELONGINGNESS
_____

SAFETY
_____

BASIC NEEDS
_____

APPRECIATION OF WORK DONE

Every year, more and more hospitals are developing experimental primary nursing systems. This approach allows the nurse to care totally for six to seven patients. Nurses have a need to know their patients as people, a need to talk with them about how they feel. The nurse must feel that the work being done is important and appreciated.

This desire to be a part of the health care team seems to permeate high-performance hospitals. A hospital dietician stated it this way: "I'm not a glorified cook. I'm a part of the health care team. The dietician and the endocrinologist working together with a diabetic patient. If this diabetic is well managed and adheres to his or her diet, then the patient may not need insulin."

The perceptions of health care employees are extremely important. Whatever they believe to be true is true for them. If they feel they are a part of a "team," they are indeed a part of a team. Individuals can respond to appreciation of work done only in terms of their perceptions. Therefore, the result of communication between supervisor and subordinate will be what the subordinate perceives it to be.

FEELING IN ON THINGS

Nurses at times become irked at the indifference of doctors to nurses' opinions about patients. As one nurse put it, "Sometimes you

wonder why you have to make the rounds with an M.D., when he totally ignores your questions and suggestions."

W.C. Redding found that "good communication" characterizes effective managerial leadership:[3]

1. The better supervisors tend to be communication-minded, are
able to explain instructions and policies, and enjoy conversing with
subordinates.

2. The better supervisors tend to be empathic listeners; they respond understandingly to "silly" questions; they are approachable;
they will listen to suggestions and complaints with an attitude of
fair consideration and a willingness to take appropriate action.

3. The better supervisors tend to ask or persuade rather than tell or
demand.

4. The better supervisors tend to be sensitive to the feelings and
ego-defense needs of their subordinates; they are careful to reprimand in private rather than in public.

5. The better supervisors openly pass along information; they give
advance notice of impending changes and supply "reasons" for
policies and regulations.

When nurses are not involved in the decision-making process and are
rarely consulted, there is a tendency to let down and not be totally involved in the job. The result of such indifference is job dissatisfaction.
It follows that, if nurses feel they are not wisely utilized, it is next to
impossible to instill any degree of pride into their work. High job
satisfaction and quality patient care depend upon the maximum use of
the individual's training and skill.

At times, fear is also used as a motivator. Sometimes people are
called in and told, "Look, if this doesn't stop, we are going to see some
new faces around here." However, this can be only a temporary solution. The best solution is to call people together and say, "What can we
do to improve this situation?" People can be motivated only through
the sharing of power and not through the exertion of power by one individual. If there is a nursing problem, rather than one individual trying to solve it, what better solution is there than to call the group
together to share ideas. No one knows the job better than the nurse
who is doing it day in and day out.

F.B. Chaney discovered that there was a positive correlation between performance and job attitude and the degree of participation in
the decision-making process. He reported zero improvement for people
in no-participation to low-participation groups, while the high-

participation groups showed an attitude and production improvement of 80 percent and 95 percent respectively.[4]

PROFESSIONAL GROWTH

Work must be a source of personal enrichment, and nurses must feel that they have an opportunity to grow and become the professionals they are capable of becoming. Participating in in-house training programs, attending conventions, and belonging to professional organizations help the nurse fulfill the needs of self-actualization. Quality care depends upon internal growth within a hospital, but this growth is dependent in turn upon the personal growth of the hospital's employees.

Frederick Herzberg examined factors affecting job attitudes. He tallied 1,844 events on the job that, when absent, led to extreme dissatisfaction; he labeled these events maintenance factors. He also tallied 1,753 events on the job that led to extreme satisfaction, and these he called motivators.

Herzberg, like Maslow, found that motivational needs are not mutually exclusive and that indeed one need may build upon another. Also, people may be motivated by several needs at the same time.

Herzberg rank ordered the following motivators and maintenance factors by their percentage of frequency:[5]

Motivators	Maintenance Factors
Extreme Satisfaction	Extreme Dissatisfaction
1. Achievement	1. Company Policy and Administration
2. Recognition	2. Supervision
3. Work Itself	3. Relationship with Supervisor
4. Responsibility	4. Work Conditions
5. Advancement	5. Salary
6. Growth	6. Relationship with Peers

Remember that the maintenance factors created job dissatisfaction only when they were lacking or absent from the job. If employees are involved in the decision-making process, are allowed to have job input along with an opportunity to improve their skills, these factors can prevent dissatisfaction and poor job performance.

CHALLENGING WORK

More than ever before, nurses are concerned about two themes: (1) concern that the job be a source of personal fulfillment, and (2) the right to assert individual rights on the job, sometimes called "the psychology of entitlement." When nurses feel that they are a part of a team working toward a common goal, their level of personal fulfillment will be raised. When their questions and suggestions are listened to, their individual rights as a professional are maintained. Today, values are shifting in the nursing profession. The baby-boom children who came into the job force in the late sixties and early seventies account for this new youthfulness. Nurses under 30 years of age are demanding that a job be both interesting and challenging. Older nurses are now starting to express the same sentiment. They want to feel that nursing is more than just a job. They want to feel that what they do matters. There is a greater demand to be heard and to be involved in the decision-making process.

The importance of job satisfaction is starting to permeate all vocations. In a national survey of newly licensed nurses conducted by the Department of Health, Education, and Welfare in 1975, it was found that many nurses currently employed in one type of institution would actually have preferred another type of employer:[6]

Job Dissatisfaction

Present Employer	% Preferring Another Type of Employer	1st Choice of Another Employer
Public Hospital	22%	Private Hospital
Private Hospital	33	Public Hospital
Nursing Home	67	Public Hospital

Source: Department of Health, Education, and Welfare, May, 1975.

The study also reported that 51 percent of the newly licensed nurses felt their skills were wisely utilized, but this feeling was not shared by graduates of baccalaureate programs. It was found that 40 percent of the baccalaureate graduates—a greater percentage than in any other type of nursing program—reported that their skills were underutilized.[7]

Another nursing survey, conducted in 1975, asked the question, "What aspects of your job do you find most dissatisfying?" Some typical responses were:[8]

- I thoroughly enjoy my job and my coworkers. If we were adequately staffed, I could tolerate anything.
- You make plans and then something goes wrong, and there goes your day off.
- I have the responsibility, yes, but not the authority to do the job.
- I have very little opportunity for continuing education.

In a national survey conducted by *Nursing 76* on job dissatisfaction among nurses, it was discovered that 44 percent were dissatisfied with their jobs. At the same time, 46 percent were satisfied, and 10 percent failed to reply.[9]

The above comments, along with the statistical data, seem to indicate that today it takes more than just money and security to motivate nurses. The motivational needs of people are changing as rapidly as technology, and these needs must be met.

GOOD WAGES

Few nurses enter the profession for the financial rewards it offers. However, to be a profession, it must pay like a profession. Money in any vocation can motivate people. Money will initially attract people to a particular career, but most motivational theorists will tell you that money is not a long-lasting motivator. For example, only a minority of nurses are dissatisfied with their incomes. When nurses are dissatisfied, the reasons go deeper than a low salary. It could be a lack of praise for a job well done, humiliation at the hands of a doctor, demeaning supervision, or inability to participate in the decision-making process.

The fact remains that as we become involved in our jobs, in the daily routine, we quickly forget that recent raise or the forthcoming raise at the end of the year. If a nurse is making a salary similar to that of another nurse in the same geographical area and with equal years of experience, money will not be a primary issue. However, if the nurse finds that other nurses in the same area with the same amount of experience are making more money, then money does become an issue.

The University of Michigan Survey Research Center asked 1,553 working people to rank order various aspects of their jobs in order of importance. The center discovered that "good pay" came in fifth behind "interesting work," "enough help and equipment to get the job done," "enough information to do the job," and "enough authority to do the job."[10]

Earlier in this chapter you were asked to rank order ten items pertaining to the needs of the health care professional. Note the similarities between that survey and the University of Michigan survey cited above.

The nurses, you will remember, were asked to rank order the items with respect to their importance to them personally. On the other hand, the nursing supervisors and hospital administrators were asked for their personal ranking along with how they thought their employees would rank the items. This was done in an attempt to determine if management had an accurate perception of what was "really" important to employees from a motivational point of view. The results, shown below, speak for themselves.

The Needs of the Health Care Professional

Your Rating		Nurses' Rating	Supervisors' Rating
_____	Appreciation of Work Done.	1	8
_____	Feeling "in" on Things.	2	10
_____	Professional Growth.	3	2
_____	Challenging Work.	4	5
_____	Good Wages.	5	1
_____	Good Working Conditions.	6	4
_____	Management Loyalty to Workers.	7	6
_____	Promotion.	8	3
_____	Help on Personal Problems.	9	9
_____	Tactful Disciplining.	10	7

Several generalizations can be made from this study. The study seems to indicate that nurses are seeking "real" involvement in their jobs and that this is what made the profession initially attractive. When nurses become less involved in direct patient care, their job-satisfaction level decreases. Consequently, they become dissatisfied with the practice setting. This dissatisfaction has resulted in nursing shortages in some hospitals. Nurse turnover and/or absenteeism result in lost revenue and, more important, in lower quality care to patients. When a nurse is absent, someone else must do the job. To eliminate this problem, it is important that an attempt be made to determine the motivational needs of the nurse.

Finally, it is much easier to communicate in a meaningful manner when we have a data base from which to draw realistic perceptions as to each other's needs. Only through congruent perceptions can we solve problems and work together toward a common goal. Too many times our perceptions of another's needs are false perceptions. For example, if money is important to us, we assume it's important to others as well. Therefore, we don't take the time or effort to seek genuine feedback. Many times hospital policy is based on inaccurate information; and, to compound the problem, when nurses are asked for feedback, they sometimes fail to be open and honest and they supply faulty information, disguising the real issues.

Many different types of instruments are used in an attempt to determine organizational and/or employee needs. The feedback information from such instruments can be used to implement new policies or, if need be, to change existing ones.

The following Motivation Feedback Questionnaire will tell you what motivates you. However, remember that, just because some of these items motivate you, that does not mean they will motivate everyone else. A popular television show a few years ago had the theme, "Different Strokes for Different Folks." In respect to motivational theory, that theme holds true.

Motivation Feedback Questionnaire

Part I

Directions:

The following statements have seven possible responses.

Strongly Agree	Agree	Slightly Agree	Don't Know	Slightly Disagree	Disagree	Strongly Disagree
+3	+2	+1	0	−1	−2	−3

Please score each statement by circling the number that corresponds to your response. For example, if you "Strongly Agree," circle the number "+3."

1. Special salary increases should be given to employees who do their jobs well. +3 +2 +1 0 −1 −2 −3

2. Better job descriptions would be helpful so that employees know exactly what is expected of them. +3 +2 +1 0 −1 −2 −3

3. Employees need to be reminded that their jobs are dependent upon the group's ability to meet its objective. +3 +2 +1 0 −1 −2 −3

4. Supervisors should give a great deal of attention to the physical working conditions of their employees. +3 +2 +1 0 −1 −2 −3

5. Supervisors ought to work hard to develop a friendly working atmosphere among their employees. +3 +2 +1 0 −1 −2 −3

6. Individual recognition for above-standard performance means a lot to employees. +3 +2 +1 0 −1 −2 −3

7. Indifferent supervision can often bruise feelings. +3 +2 +1 0 −1 −2 −3

8. Employees want to feel that their real skills and capacities are put to use on their jobs. +3 +2 +1 0 −1 −2 −3

9. The group's retirement benefits and medical insurance programs are important factors in keeping employees on their jobs. +3 +2 +1 0 −1 −2 −3

10. Almost every job can be made more stimulating and challenging. +3 +2 +1 0 −1 −2 −3

11. Many employees want to give their best in everything they do.   +3 +2 +1 0 −1 −2 −3

12. Management could show more interest in the employees by sponsoring social events after hours.   +3 +2 +1 0 −1 −2 −3

13. Pride in one's work is actually an important reward.   +3 +2 +1 0 −1 −2 −3

14. Employees want to think of themselves as the "best" at their jobs.   +3 +2 +1 0 −1 −2 −3

15. The quality of the relationships in the informal work group is quite important.   +3 +2 +1 0 −1 −2 −3

16. Individual merit raises would improve the performance of employees.   +3 +2 +1 0 −1 −2 −3

17. Visibility with upper management is important to employees.   +3 +2 +1 0 −1 −2 −3

18. Employees generally like to schedule their own work and make job-related decisions with a minimum of supervision.   +3 +2 +1 0 −1 −2 −3

19. Job security is important to employees.   +3 +2 +1 0 −1 −2 −3

20. Having good equipment to work with is important to employees.   +3 +2 +1 0 −1 −2 −3

Part II

SCORING:

1. Enter the numbers you circled in Part I in the blanks below after the appropriate statement number.

STATEMENT NO.	SCORE	STATEMENT NO.	SCORE
10	_____	2	_____
11	_____	3	_____
13	_____	9	_____
18	_____	19	_____
SELF-ACTUALIZATION_____TOTAL		SAFETY_____TOTAL	

STATEMENT NO.	SCORE
6	____
8	____
14	____
17	____

ESTEEM____TOTAL

STATEMENT NO.	SCORE
1	____
4	____
16	____
20	____

BASIC____TOTAL

STATEMENT NO.	SCORE
5	____
7	____
12	____
15	____

BELONGINGNESS____TOTAL

2. Record your scores in the chart below by putting an "X" in each row under the number of your total score for that area of need-motivation.

Once you have completed this chart, you can see the relative strength of your response in each area of "need-motivation." There is of course no "right" answer. What motivates you might not motivate someone else. In general, however, most motivational theorists believe that most employees are motivated by managers who stress the belongingness and esteem needs of their employees.

DEGREE OF EMPHASIS	-12	-10	-8	-6	-4	-2	0	+2	+4	+6	+8	+10	+12
SELF-ACTUALIZATION													
ESTEEM													
BELONGINGNESS													
SAFETY													
BASIC													

LOW USE   HIGH USE

This conclusion can be supported by recent productivity figures in Japan. The Japanese simply outmanage us when it comes to people. They view their businesses and hospitals as social organizations, not simply as profit-oriented enterprises. The Japanese believe that the most important information flows from the bottom up and not from the top down. Their managers and supervisors expect change and initiative to come from those closest to the problem rather than from the top administrators. Many American corporations are now changing to this style of management. The organizational climate in Japan is centered around humanistic psychology in which human relations are just as important as production. Ultimately, the relationships between workers and management will be reflected in the quality of the goods or services.

MOTIVATION REVIEW PUZZLE

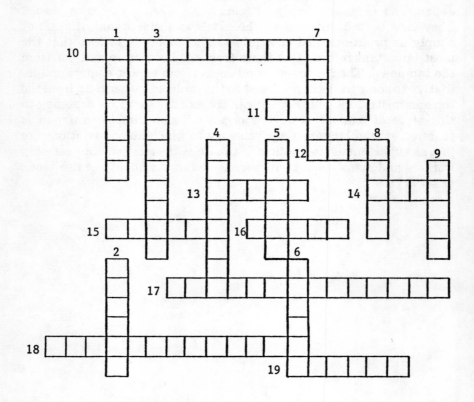

DOWN

1) A nursing system.
2) Ranked third by nurses.
3) Creates extreme satisfaction.
4) The primary concern of a hospital.
5) Developed hierarchy of human needs.
6) To respect.
7) Who's in the people business?
8) How nurses rated good wages.
9) A long lasting motivator.

ACROSS

10) Nurses rank it number one.
11) Need for food, clothing, shelter.
12) Who motivates you?
13) Improves morale.
14) Few people are motivated by this.
15) Their responses determine quality of service.
16) Is not a long lasting motivator.
17) Improves morale.
18) What decision making should be.
19) You want a high degree of this.

(Answers are on page 19.)

NOTES

1. Douglas McGregor, *The Human Side of Enterprise* (New York: McGraw-Hill Book Co., 1960), p. 6.
2. Abraham Maslow, *Motivation and Personality* (New York: Harper & Row, 1954).
3. W.C. Redding, *Communication Within the Organization* (West Lafayette, Indiana: Purdue University, Industrial Communication Council, 1972), p. 443.
4. F. B. Chaney, "Employee Participation in Manufacturing Job Design," *Human Factors* 11: 101–106.
5. Frederick Herzberg, "One More Time How Do You Motivate Employees?" *Harvard Business Review* 46, no. 1: 53–62.
6. P.M. Nash, "Evaluation of Employment Opportunities for Newly Licensed Nurses." Division of Research, National League for Nursing. Published by Health Resources Administration of HEW, May 1975, DHEW No. [HRA] 75-12, pp. 50–51.
7. *Ibid.,* p. 59.
8. Marjorie Godfrey, "Working Conditions," *Nursing 75,* May, 1975.
9. Howard S. Rowland, ed., "Job Satisfaction," *The Nurse's Almanac* (Germantown, Md.: Aspen Systems Corp., 1978), p. 101.
10. Donald M. Morrison, "Is the Work Ethic Going Out of Style?" in *The Challenge of the Future: Visions and Versions,* ed. Bill Conboy (Lawrence, Kansas: The University of Kansas, Division of Continuing Education, 1979), p. 161.

SUGGESTED READINGS

Atkinson, J.W., and Raynor, J.O. *Motivation and Achievement.* New York: Halstead Press, 1974.

Beer, M. *Leadership, Employee Needs, and Motivation.* Columbus: Bureau of Business Research, Ohio State University, 1966.

Centers, R., and Bugental, D. "Intrinsic and Extrinsic Motivations Among Different Segments of the Working Population," *Journal of Applied Psychology* 50: 193–197.

Dalton, Gene W., and Lawrence, Paul R. *Motivation and Control in Organizations.* Homewood, Illinois: Richard D. Irwin Inc., 1971.

Evans, M. "Herzberg's Two Factor Motivation: Some Problems and a Suggested Test." *Personnel Journal* 49: 32–35.

Ganong, Warren, and Ganong, Joan. "Good Advice: Motivation and Innovation—Concerns for Nursing Administration," *Journal of Nursing Administration* 3: 7–9.

Gellerman, Saul W. *Motivation and Productivity.* New York: American Management Association, 1963.

Goble, Frank. *The Third Force: The Psychology of Abraham Maslow.* New York: Grossman Publishers, 1970.

Hall, D.T., and Nougaim, K.E., "An Examination of Maslow's Need Hierarchy in An Organizational Setting," *Organizational Behavior and Human Performance* 5, no. 1: 12–35.

Herzberg, Frederick. "One More Time How Do You Motivate Employees?" *Harvard Business Review* 46, no. 1: 53–62.

House, R.J., and Wingdor, L.A., "Herzberg's Dual-Factor Theory of Job Satisfaction and Motivation," *Personnel Psychology* 20, no. 4: 369–389.

Maslow, Abraham H. *Motivation and Personality*. New York: Harper & Row, 1970.

_____. *Toward a Psychology of Being*. Princeton: Van Nostrand Insight Books, 1968.

McClelland, David C., ed. *Studies in Motivation*. New York: Appleton-Century-Crofts, 1955.

McGregor, Douglas. *Leadership and Motivation*. Edited by Warren G. Bennis and Edgar H. Schien. Cambridge, Mass.: Massachusetts Institute of Technology Press, 1966.

Moser, George V. "How Not to Influence People," *Management Record*, March, 1958.

Schneider, Frank W., and Delaney, James D. "Effect of Individual Achievement Motivation on Group Problem Solving Efficiency," *Journal of Social Psychology* 86: 291–298.

Steers, Richard M. and Porter, Lyman, W. *Motivation and Work Behavior*. New York: McGraw-Hill Book Co., 1975.

Vroom, Victor H. *Work and Motivation*. New York: John Wiley and Sons Inc., 1964.

MOTIVATION REVIEW PUZZLE

```
 1       3                    7
10 A  P  P  R  E  C  I  A  T  I  O  N
   R     E                    U
   I     C                    R
   M     O          11 B  A  S  I  C
   A     G       4        5    E        8
   R     N       P        M  12 S  E  L  F        9
   Y     I       A        A       I           P
         T  13 T  R  U  S  T    14 F  E  A  R
         I     I        L          T           I
15 P  E  O  P  L  E  16 M  O  N  E  Y  H        D
         N     N        W  6                    E
  2      G     T        E
   G
   R  17 R  E  S  P  O  N  S  I  B  I  L  I  T  Y
   O                    T
   W                    E
18 P  A  R  T  I  C  I  P  A  T  I  V  E
   H                 19 M  O  R  A  L  E
```

DOWN

1) A nursing system.
2) Ranked third by nurses.
3) Creates extreme satisfaction.
4) The primary concern of a hospital.
5) Developed hierarchy of human needs.
6) To respect.
7) Who's in the people business?
8) How nurses rated good wages.
9) A long lasting motivator.

ACROSS

10) Nurses rank it number one.
11) Need for food, clothing, shelter.
12) Who motivates you?
13) Improves morale.
14) Few people are motivated by this.
15) Their responses determine quality of service.
16) Is not a long lasting motivator.
17) Improves morale.
18) What decision making should be.
19) You want a high degree of this.

Chapter 2

The Nurse as an Organizational Climate Maker

CHAPTER OBJECTIVES

> The purpose of this chapter is to enable you to CHANGE your communicative behavior in a *positive* direction. After studying the material you should be able to:
>
> **C** omprehend the importance of organizational climate.
>
> **H** elp your work group improve its organizational climate.
>
> **A** nalyze the existing organizational climate in your work group.
>
> **N** otice the effects of organizational climate on patient care.
>
> **G** uide your work group toward greater group cohesion.
>
> **E** xamine your role as a climate maker.

What is organizational climate? Can it be used to motivate and enhance the performance of workers? The dimensions of an organizational climate seem to vary from theorist to theorist, but the combined research seems to suggest that various small group variables determine the organizational climate of a group.

William Evans defined organizational climate as "a multidimensional perception by members, as well as nonmembers, of the essential attributes or character of an organizational system."[1]

There are certain properties that may be classified as attributes that help form the character of an organization. These attributes or properties play an instrumental role in developing group climate.

Dorwin Cartwright has identified nine group properties that appear to have potential value, depending upon the motives of the people involved:[2]

1. attractiveness of group members
2. similarities among members
3. nature of group goals
4. type of interdependence among group members
5. activities of the group
6. style of leadership and the opportunity to participate in decisions
7. various structural properties of the group
8. the group atmosphere
9. size of the group

Evans makes the following "assumptions" about organizational climate:[3]

- Members as well as nonmembers have perceptions of the climate of the organization.
- Organizational members tend to perceive the climate differently from nonmembers because of the prevalence of different frames of reference and different criteria for evaluating an organization.
- Perceptions of organizational climate, whether real or unreal, have behavorial consequences for the organization as well as for elements of the organization-set, i.e., the complement of organizations with which the organization interacts.
- Organizational members performing differing roles tend to have different perceptions of the climate, if only because of (1) a lack of role consensus, (2) a lack of uniformity in role socialization, and (3) a diversity in patterns of role-set interactions.

- Members of different organizational subunits tend to have different perceptions of the climate because of different role-set configurations, different subgoals, and a differential subcommitment to the goals of subunits compared to the goals of the organization as a whole.

As further clarification, Andrew Halpin offers the following metaphorical description of organizational climate:

> Anyone who visits more than a few schools notes quickly how schools differ from each other in their "feel." In one school the teachers and students are zestful and exude confidence in what they are doing. They find pleasure in working with each other; this pleasure is transmitted to the students, who thus are given at least a fighting chance to discover that school can be a happy experience. In a second school the brooding discontent of the teachers is palpable; the principal tries to hide his incompetence and his lack of sense of direction behind a cloak of authority, and yet he wears this cloak poorly because the attitude he displays to others vacillates randomly between the obsequious and the officious. And the psychological sickness of such a faculty spills over on the students who, in their own frustration, feed back to the teachers a mood of despair. A third school is neither marked by joy nor despair, but by hollow ritual. Here one gets the feeling of watching an elaborate charade in which teachers, principal, and students are acting out parts. The acting is smooth, even glib, but it appears to have little meaning for the participants; in a strange way the show just doesn't seem to be "for real." And so, too, as one moves to other schools, one finds that each appears to have a "personality" of its own. It is this personality that we describe here as organizational climate of the school.[4]

We could easily substitute hospital, clinic, nursing home, or any other type of health care facility for the word "school" in the preceding metaphorical description of organizational climate. In fact, you could walk through your own facility and find unique, but obvious, differences in the organizational climates of subgroups.

THE NURSE AS A CLIMATE MAKER

What is organizational climate in a health care setting? This question can be answered best in terms of an analogy. Organizational climate is both similar to and different from the weather. For example, more than 20 percent of the American population watches the weather report each night to find out what the weather will be like the next day. In another context, the climate affects our relationships with people. Doesn't the behavior of people toward one another seem to be different on a clear, bright, 70-degree Spring day compared to a stormy, 10-degree day with sleet and snow?

Considerable evidence seems to indicate that, just as people tend to take cues on clothing and behavior from the weather, they are also influenced by the kind of organizational climate within a hospital. The organizational climate affects the behavior of the hospital's administrators, aides, technicians, doctors, nurses, and patients.

At this point, however, the analogy ends, and the differences between the weather and organizational climate begin to appear. Unlike the weather, the organizational climate of a hospital is not something that we can directly see or touch. We can nevertheless sense it just as easily as a nurse or physician can sense that something is wrong with a patient. Though no thermometer can measure it, the organizational climate can be manipulated and changed. The real weather of wind, rain, and snow cannot be changed and goes its merry way. But people create their own work environment; if it isn't right, people can change it.

Numerous studies have shown that certain types of climates typify high performance groups. The recent move back to primary nursing indicates that climate making can influence how nurses feel about their work. The resulting feelings are then transmitted into hard realities, such as individual motivation and effort, goal clarity, group cohesiveness, and a continuing commitment to goals.

No matter how many positive factors—such as good planning by hospital administrators and health care knowledge—there are within a hospital, many of the pitfalls encountered by the hospital in getting the job done will involve human problems, and such problems relate to bottom line performance, that is, excellent patient care.

The behavior a nurse exhibits on the job helps to determine the organizational climate. The combined behaviors of all health care professionals determine the "total" organizational climate of the hospital.

By exhibiting "positive" communicative behaviors nurses can:

- make their work group more cohesive,
- help others to motivate themselves,
- improve the organizational climate, and
- create a balance between the pressures for high short-term performance and the development of individual talents of the people they work with.

K.W. Back discovered that highly cohesive groups tended to place more value on communication than groups of low cohesion. The highly cohesive groups also had more communicative balance among their members. No one member seemed to dominate the thinking of the group.[5]

DIMENSIONS OF CLIMATE

There are six climate dimensions that can be categorized into two groups: (1) Performance Dimensions and (2) Development Dimensions. Through an understanding of these dimensions of climate and by applying them to their jobs, nurses can increase their effectiveness as motivational agents.

Performance Dimensions

Clarity

Clarity refers to the nurse's sense of understanding of the hospital's goals and policies. This requires an effort to make things run smoothly, as opposed to an acceptance of confusion. Nurses will change the organizational climate in a positive direction if

- they understand what is expected of them,
- they help plan and organize activities, and
- they help to see that information flows smoothly.

Commitment

Nurses must have a continuing commitment to goal achievement (patient care). This commitment is related to an acceptance of realistic goals, an involvement in goal setting, and a continuous evaluation of performance compared with the goals. Nurses will change the organizational climate in a positive direction if

- they are involved in goal setting and review meetings,
- they recognize the goals and consider them to be meaningful and realistic, and
- they have a personal commitment to achieve the goals.

Cartwright has stated that "the greater the group's cohesion the more power it has to bring about conformity to its norms and to gain acceptance of its goals and assignment to tasks and roles."[6]

Standards

Here the focus is on the emphasis that nurses place on setting high standards of performance. Nurses will change the organizational climate in a positive direction if

- they are interested in improving their performance,
- they have pride in doing a good job, and
- they set tough and challenging personal goals.

Alvin Zander found that a group's aspiration level helped to determine its degree of success or failure

> After repeated success, members who perceive that the future promises a greater likelihood of success at that level of difficulty, raise their anticipated level of aspiration, develop feelings of success and pride in the group, assign a favorable evaluation to their group's performance, attribute greater value to future success, develop a disposition to seek further success, perceive their group to be an attractive one, and become committed to the process of setting future goals. Individuals who have more responsible positions are more likely to have the reactions just described than are those with less important roles.
> On the other hand, after repeated failure, members are less inclined to be concerned about the probabilities of future failure, or success; instead, they seek means that will help them to avoid the unfavorable consequences of failure. They tend to: lower the group's goal or stick with the one they have failed to reach, give an unapproving evaluation to their group's performance, see the activity as less important, believe that success on the task is less desirable, are

less attracted to their own group, and would like to judge the group in relation to its past performance rather than its goal attainment. They would gladly abandon altogether the practice of setting aspiration levels. Members of such groups have a distinct preference for unreasonably difficult tasks, in the light of their past performance, making them highly vulnerable to subsequent failure.[7]

Development Dimensions

Responsibility

This dimension concerns the nurse's feelings of personal responsibility for work, involving both a sense of autonomy stemming from real delegation and encouragement of fellow nurses to take individual initiative. Nurses will change the organizational climate in a positive direction if

- they feel they can help others solve problems,
- they develop a sense of independence and feel their judgment is trusted, and
- they encourage themselves and others to take increased responsibility.

Cartwright discovered that members of cohesive groups more readily exert influence over one another and are more readily influenced by one another, compared to members of non-cohesive groups.[8]

Recognition

Nurses must feel that they will be recognized for doing a good job. They should not feel that criticism is more likely than recognition for good performance. Nurses will change the organizational climate in a positive direction if

- they see rewards and recognition outweighing threats and criticism,
- they see the existence of a promotion system that helps the best person to rise to the top, and
- they see rewards related to excellence of performance.

J.W. Thibaut and H.H. Kelley discovered that a person will join a group based on personal expected outcomes.

When joining a group a person employs a standard called the comparison level, against which they compare the expected outcomes of membership. This comparison level derives from their previous experience in groups and indicates the level of outcomes they aspire to receive from membership. They will be more attracted to the group the more the level of expected outcomes exceeds their comparison level.[9]

Teamwork

Nurses must feel that they belong to a health care team. This feeling is characterized by cohesion, mutual warmth and support, trust, and pride. Nurses will change the organizational climate in a positive direction if

- they see evidence of mutual understanding and support,
- they see people trusting and respecting others, and
- they develop a feeling of personal loyalty and a sense of belonging to their work group and patients.

Renis Likert found that group morale and team spirit increased when

The leadership and other processes of the organization ensure a maximum probability that in all interactions and in all relationships with the organization members will, in the light of their background, values, and expectations, view the experience as supportive and one which builds and maintains their sense of personal worth and importance.[10]

The key to Likert's conclusions is in the role of trust. High trust tends to stimulate high performance and increase employee confidence, loyalty, and teamwork.[11]

The decision to spend time improving the organizational climate within a hospital is one that nurses must make for themselves. Each nurse has a responsibility to encourage others in individual or joint efforts. Highly motivated individuals tend to work in supportive organizational climates. But it should be remembered that people make the climate. We live in climates of our own making, and these self-made climates affect our relationships with others.

A supportive climate carries into each and every room of a hospital. No one can see it or touch it, but every health care practitioner and patient can "sense" it. When nurses sense a supportive organizational climate, it reaffirms their basic reason for being, for caring about people and improved patient care.

A NURSING CLIMATE SURVEY

The following nursing climate survey is aimed at gaining a better understanding of the kind of work climate or environment in which the nurse works, of the way in which the climate is created, and how it affects job performance and ultimately the job satisfaction of the nurse.

As you fill out the questionnaire, respond to the items as they relate to your work group. Do not assume that pay, money, or economic gains are implied by any of the questions. That is, questions that deal with recognition assume nonfinancial recognition.

PART I

For each of the statements below please draw a circle around one of the following:

A — Always
F — Frequently
O — Occasionally
S — Seldom
N — Never

For example, if you feel that you are frequently encouraged to come up with new and original ideas, you would circle the "F" in the following question:

A Ⓕ O S N   1. We are encouraged to come up with new and original ideas.

Please use only one evaluative letter code for each answer.

A F O S N   1. I have the opportunity to review my overall performance and effectiveness with my supervisor.

A F O S N   2. There is much respect between management and other personnel in this group.

A F O S N   3. In this organization, the rewards and encouragements you receive for effective performance outweigh the threats and criticisms.

A F O S N   4. Our people are encouraged to make decisions when the situation demands an immediate decision.

A F O S N   5. In this group, I am given a chance to participate in setting the performance goals for my job.

A F O S N   6. People in our group are aware of what good performance means in their jobs.

A F O S N   7. I feel that I am a member of a well-functioning team.

A F O S N   8. In this group we are rewarded in proportion to how well we do our jobs.

A F O S N   9. We are encouraged to come up with new and original ideas.

A F O S N   10. Management works with us in developing challenging team and group goals.

A F O S N   11. In this group, performance is evaluated against agreed-upon performance goals.

A F O S N   12. In my group, high performers are recognized by their supervisor for their superior performance.

A F O S N   13. In this group, what constitutes good performance has been identified.

A F O S N   14. In this group, people demonstrate strong commitment to achieving performance goals.

A F O S N   15. Things seem to be fairly well organized in my group.

A F O S N   16. People in this group help each other in solving job-related problems.

A F O S N   17. My supervisor does a good job in recognizing good performance.

A F O S N   18. My supervisor emphasizes that people in this group should personally accept the responsibility for solving day-to-day operational problems.

A F O S N   19. In this group, we are encouraged to improve continually our personal and group performance.

A F O S N   20. The results I am supposed to achieve in my job are realistic.

A F O S N   21. The policies and structure of this group have been clearly explained.

A F O S N   22. People are proud to belong to this group.

A F O S N   23. In my group, very high standards are set for performance.

A F O S N   24. I am involved in setting my own performance goals and in understanding how they relate to the overall goals of my group.

A F O S N   25. The assignments in my group are clearly defined and logically structured.

If your responses were in the "always" or "frequently" columns, you see your work group in a very positive way. On the other hand, if most of your responses were "seldom" or "never," you see your group in a very negative way, and this can affect your morale.

Working conditions and an employee's perceptions of those conditions affect individual morale and determine the work climate. If the organizational climate of a hospital is not right, can a nurse change that climate? Can a nurse become a motivational agent of change? Remember, organizational climate does not just happen. Rather it is the "collective" view of the people within an organization as to the nature of the environment in which they work, and they can make that climate anything they want it to be.

CLIMATE REVIEW PUZZLE

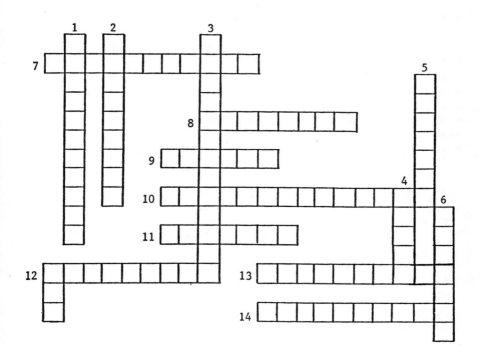

DOWN

1) A major climate dimension.
2) Determines organizational climate.
3) Affected by organizational climate.
4) Number of performance dimensions.
5) A performance dimension.
6) Similar to but different from organizational climate.

ACROSS

7) A major climate dimension.
8) A development dimension.
9) Who creates organizational climate?
10) A development dimension.
11) A collective organizational view.
12) A performance dimension.
13) Another performance dimension.
14) Highly motivated individuals tend to work in _____ organizational climates.

(Answers are on page 36.)

NOTES

1. William Evans, *Organizational Theory: Structures, Systems, and Environment* (New York: John Wiley and Sons, 1976), p. 137.

2. Dorwin Cartwright, "The Nature of Group Cohesiveness," in *Group Dynamics*, ed. D. Cartwright and A. Zander (New York: Harper & Row, 1968), p. 107.

3. Evans, *Organizational Theory*, p. 139.

4. Andrew Halpin, *Theory and Research in Administration* (New York: Macmillan and Co., 1966), p. 131.

5. K.W. Back, "Influence Through Social Communication," *Journal of Social Psychology* 46: 9-23.

6. Cartwright, "Nature of Group Cohesiveness," p. 91.

7. Alvin Zander, *Motives and Goals in Groups* (New York:Academic Press, Inc. 1971), p. 174.

8. Cartwright, "Nature of Group Cohesiveness," p. 104.

9. J.W. Thibaut and H.H. Kelley, *The Social Psychology of Groups* (New York: Wiley, 1959), p. 98.

10. Renis Likert, *New Patterns in Management* (New York: McGraw-Hill Book Co., 1961), p. 103.

11. _____, *The Human Organization* (New York: McGraw-Hill Book Co., 1967), pp. 4-10.

SUGGESTED READINGS

Exline, R. "Group Climate as a Factor in the Relevance and Accuracy of Social Perception." *Journal of Abnormal and Social Psychology* 55: 382-388.

Guion, R.M. "A Note on Organizational Climate." *Organizational Behavior and Human Performance* 9: 120-125.

James, L.R., and Jones, Allen P. "Organizational Climate: A Review of Theory and Research." *Psychological Bulletin* 81, no. 12: 1096-1112.

Johannesson, R.E. "Some Problems in the Measurement of Organizational Climate." *Organizational Behavior and Human Performance* 10: 118-144.

Kehoe, P.T., and Reddin, R. *Organizational Health Survey*. Fredericton, N.B., Canada: Organizational Tests Limited.

LaFollette, W.R., and Sims, H.P. "Is Satisfaction Redundant With Climate?" *Organizational Behavior and Human Performance* 13: 252-278.

Lawler, E.E.; Hall, Douglas T.; and Oldham, Greg R. "Organizational Climate: Relationship to Organizational Structure, Process, and Performance." *Organizational Behavior and Human Performance* 11: 139-155.

Lee, C. "Organizational Climate: A Laboratory Approach." Master's thesis, Department of Communication, Ohio State University, 1975.

Litwin, G., and Stringer, R. *Motivation and Organizational Climate*. Boston: Harvard University Press, 1967.

Lott, A., and Lott, B. "Group Cohesiveness, Communication Level, and Conformity." *Journal of Abnormal and Social Psychology* 62: 408-412.

Pepitone, A., and Reichling, G. "Group Cohesiveness and the Expression of Hostility." *Human Relations* 8: 327–343.

Perrow, C. "Hospitals: Technology, Structure, and Goals." In *Handbook of Organizations,* edited by J. March, Chapter 8. Chicago: Rand McNally, 1965.

Pritchard, R.D., and Karasick, B. "The Effect of Organizational Climate on Managerial Job Attitudes and Job Satisfaction." *Organizational Behavior and Human Performance* 9: 126–146.

Raven, B., and Rietsema, J. "The Effect of Varied Clarity of Group Goal and Group Path Upon the Individual and His Relationship to His Group." *Human Relations* 10: 29–44.

Van Zelst, R. "Sociometrically Selected Work Teams Increase Production." *Personnel Psychology* 5: 175–186.

Willerman, B., and Swanson, L. "Group Prestige in Voluntary Organization." *Human Relations* 6: 57–77.

CLIMATE REVIEW PUZZLE

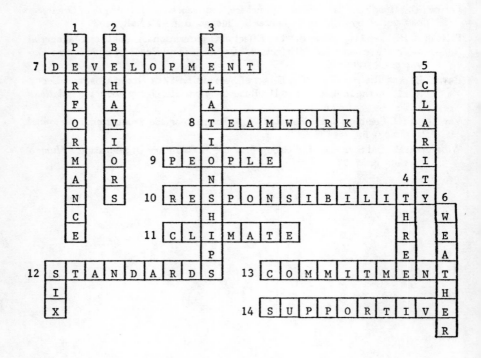

DOWN

1) A major climate dimension.
2) Determines organizational climate.
3) Affected by organizational climate.
4) Number of performance dimensions.
5) A performance dimension.
6) Similar to but different from organizational climate.

ACROSS

7) A major climate dimension.
8) A development dimension.
9) Who creates organizational climate?
10) A development dimension.
11) A collective organizational view.
12) A performance dimension.
13) Another performance dimension.
14) Highly motivated individuals tend to work in _____ organizational climates.

Chapter 3

Improved Patient Care through Deliberative Listening

CHAPTER OBJECTIVES

The purpose of this chapter is to enable you to CHANGE your communicative behavior in a *positive* direction. After studying the material you should be able to:

Communicate more effectively through the development of good listening habits.
Heighten your ability to understand other people through better listening.
Assess your listening ability.
Name and apply appropriate listening responses.
Gain the belief that listening can be improved.
Eradicate poor listening habits.

One of our first experiences with education was the first day we were sent off to school. One of the exciting times in this period of our lives was when we were told to bring an object to class and tell the class about it. This may have been our first experience with public speaking. The following years were devoted to endless classes in reading, writing, and arithmetic; but probably one of the most important of all skills was overlooked—the art of listening.

Bill Conboy has said that listening is a skill. Listening proficiency can be improved with practice. It is not a static condition like the shape of your nose or feet. Research in both business and education has demonstrated that most individuals can improve in listening performance.[1]

Warren Ganong of the Methods Engineering Council compared trainees who had knowledge of listening skills to those who had no knowledge. Those with listening-skill knowledge achieved marks 12 to 15 percent higher than those with no knowledge.[2]

Many employees in industry and business today feel they are paid to "do" a job, that a job requires "doing." However, they overlook the importance that listening plays in "doing" a job well. Listening can mean greater efficiency. Listening stems from the need to gather necessary data. Listening helps in settling grievances. Listening makes people feel special.

Many companies are recognizing the value of effective listening and have added courses in listening to their training programs. A few of these companies are American Telephone and Telegraph, General Motors Corporation, The Dow Chemical Company, Minnesota Mining and Manufacturing, and Western Electric.

DELIBERATIVE LISTENING

Charles Kelly has defined deliberative listening as a unitary skill, the ability to hear information, to analyze it, to recall it at a later time, and to draw conclusions from it. In deliberative listening, one strives to understand the message for the purpose of using the information contained in the message.[3]

Listening Requires Time and Effort

Although, in the form of "self-talk," we spend a great deal of time listening to ourselves, at times we don't even do that well. About 70 percent of our working day is spent in verbal communication. Research shows that average working adults divide their communication time roughly along these lines:[4]

Listening	45%
Talking	30%
Reading	16%
Writing	9%

These statistics indicate that almost one-half of our communication time is spent in listening. A failure to listen not only affects the relationships between doctors and nurses, but also their relationships with their patients. Before reading further, think carefully and write down your own personal definition of the word "communication." How you define that word will tell you something about you as a listener.

At the fifth annual Hospital Topics Nursing Conference, held in 1977 in Dallas, nurses were asked to write down their personal definition of the word "communication." Some of those in attendance defined communication as the process of sending messages. This definition emphasized the sending aspect of communication and overlooked the importance of the need for a receiver (listener). Just because a message was sent does not mean it was received or listened to. To have good communication, someone must take the time and effort to listen to and understand what has been said. The health care professional who defines communication simply as the process of sending messages might be inclined to say

- "I'm the doctor, and I don't have time for a lot of silly questions," or
- "I told the patient what I meant; why can't he understand that."

Other nurses at the conference defined communication as the process of sending *and* receiving messages. They understood that in order to have good communication there must be deliberative listening that evolves into interaction, exchange of information, and understanding. These respondents focused on the receiving or listening aspects of the communicative act.

When something is extremely important, there is a need for a communication check. The nurse must find out if the message was listened to. Was it received the way it was intended to be received? Was there a transfer of common meaning? The health care professional that is concerned with communication in this manner might say,

- "To answer the nurses' questions, I have to listen to what is being asked;"
- "Good communication is when I understand what the patient has said;" or
- "Communication is effective when I listen to what my nurses have to say and when they listen to what I have to say."

Your personal definition of communication, which you have written down, expresses your attitude toward the listening aspect of communication. If you defined communication with emphasis on the receiving end as well as the sending end, you recognized the importance of listening.

Upon closer examination, we discover that it is the listening side of the communicative act that enables us to gather the necessary data to solve problems, to settle a grievance, to become more efficient, to build a supportive climate, or to make a person feel special. During examinations, the doctor and nurse do not tell patients how they should feel. The patient sends messages and the doctor and nurse receive feedback through listening. By this we are not referring to a situation in which someone has you for dinner and two weeks later you have them over for a "feedback." The term "feedback" refers rather to the "certified mail" of communication. It enables one to make sure the information was received the way it was intended to be received.

Listening Responses

One of the deceptive features of listening behavior stems from our comparative lack of feedback with respect to how we are doing. A listening response is a very brief comment or action made to another person to convey the idea that the recipient is interested, attentive and wants the person to continue. The response is made quietly and briefly, so as not to interfere with the speaker's train of thought. It is usually made when the speaker pauses. There are five types of listening responses:

Nod:	Nodding the head slightly and waiting.
Pause:	Looking at the speaker expectantly.
Casual Remark:	"I see." "Uh-huh." "Is that right?"
Query:	Asking genuine questions.
Paraphrasing:	Repeating back to the speaker your understanding of what has been said.

Can improved listening skills improve not only your own ability to listen but also the ability of others to listen? In this area, common sense tells us that no one can force others to do something they don't want to do. The most that you can hope for is that your behavior will act as a model for others to emulate. A particular kind of behavior normally brings about a like behavior. If you listen to someone, there is at least the possibility that that person will also listen to you.

HOW DO YOU RATE AS A LISTENER?

Take the following test and see how you rate as a listener. Place an "X" in the appropriate blank. When speaking interpersonally with a patient, nursing supervisor, doctor, or coworker, do you:

Usually	Sometimes	Seldom	
_____	_____	_____	(1) Prepare yourself physically by standing or sitting, facing the speaker, and making sure you can hear?
_____	_____	_____	(2) Watch the speaker for the verbal as well as the nonverbal messages?
_____	_____	_____	(3) Decide from the speaker's appearance and delivery whether or not what he or she has to say is worthwhile?
_____	_____	_____	(4) Listen primarily for ideas and underlying feelings?
_____	_____	_____	(5) Determine your own bias, if any, and try to allow for it?
_____	_____	_____	(6) Keep your mind on what the speaker is saying?
_____	_____	_____	(7) Interrupt immediately if you hear a statement you feel is wrong?
_____	_____	_____	(8) Try to see the situation from the other person's point of view?
_____	_____	_____	(9) Try to have the last word?

(10) Make a conscientious effort to evaluate the logic
and credibility of what
you hear?

_____ _____ _____

SCORING

This check list, though by no means complete, should help you measure your listening ability. Score yourself as follows: Questions 1, 2, 4, 5, 6, 8, and 10—ten points for *usually,* five points for *sometimes,* and zero points for *seldom.* Questions 3, 7, and 9—zero points for *usually,* five points for *sometimes,* and ten points for *seldom.*

If you scored below 70, your listening skills can be improved because you have developed some undesirable listening habits; 70 to 85, you listen well but can still improve; 90 or above, you are an excellent listener.

People tend to do things well when they hold positive views or "labels" about their ability to do it. You can't do it until you think you can. There is a human tendency to live up or down to labels. If you think you are a good listener, you probably are, and, because of this positive label, you make a conscientious effort to listen, to live up to your label. If you say you are a poor listener, you have turned off your listening mechanism. You must think you can do it before you attempt to do it. If you fail to try because of your fear of failure, you may never discover your hidden potential.

At a recent workshop, a nurse approached the author after taking a tape-recorded listening test and remarked, "If I hadn't done well on that test I would have been very disappointed, because I consider myself to be an excellent listener." In other words, she scored as an excellent listener, and her positive attitude toward listening played a key role in her listening effectiveness.

CHECKLIST OF GUIDELINES TO IMPROVE LISTENING SKILLS

The following guidelines, in conjunction with the test you just took, should provide a more comprehensive basis to improve your listening skills:

1. You should prepare yourself physically by standing or facing the speaker. Making sure you can hear physically is essential for good listening. You thereby tell the sender that you are ready to listen

and are able to hear the verbal messages and also see the nonverbal messages the speaker is sending. This face-to-face attention also shows that you are interested in what is being said. People tend to avoid and look away from people and things in which they are not interested. Attention and interest are synonymous. You pay attention to the things you are interested in, and you are interested in the things you pay attention to.

2. You should learn to watch for the speaker's nonverbal as well as verbal messages. Everyone sends two messages. One message is sent verbally and the other is sent nonverbally through inflection in the voice or through facial expression, bodily action, or gestures. Sixty-eight percent of all messages are sent nonverbally. The nonverbal message conveys the speaker's attitude, sincerity, and genuineness. To miss the nonverbal message is to miss half of what is being said.

3. You should not decide from the speaker's appearance or delivery that what he or she has to say is worthwhile. When you start to focus on the speaker's delivery or appearance, you become distracted from the purpose of communication, receiving the speaker's ideas! You should be more interested in what people have to say than how they say it or what they look like.

4. You should listen for ideas and underlying feelings. Again, the purpose of good communication is to be able to reflect upon and exchange ideas. For example, if I were to meet you on the street and give you a dollar and you gave me a dollar, and you then went your way and I went mine, neither of us would be better off because of the exchange. But if I gave you an idea and you gave me an idea, then both of us would be better off as a result of the exchange.

5. You should try to determine your own biases, if any, and allow for them. Communication gets blamed for many things. Whenever something doesn't go right, you might say you have a communication breakdown. But many times you don't have a communication breakdown at all. In fact, you might have very good communication; you both know what has been said, and there is a common understanding. But you don't like what you have heard. If the nurse, physician, or surgeon could learn to recognize such differences, better relationships would be formed. You will not always agree with everyone. The trauma in such situations develops when you discover you are no longer talking about the issues, but about each other.

6. You should attempt to keep your mind on what the speaker is saying. Don't allow yourself to become distracted. Too many times peo-

ple fake attention and like the little dog in the back of the car window just keep nodding their heads up and down without hearing a word of what is being said.

7. You should not interrupt immediately if you hear a statement that you feel is wrong. Indeed, if you listen closely, you may be persuaded that the statement is right. Sometimes you may fail to listen just because of this fear of something different, of the possibility that you may have to forsake some sacred position you have held for years.

8. You should try to see the situation from the other person's point of view. This doesn't mean that you always have to agree. However, there is no way that you can change other people's perceptions until you can see how they have formulated those perceptions.

9. You should not try to have the last word. Listen to what is being said and then think about it. This reflection may take some time, but you need time to think before you communicate. Sometimes, in order to solve problems, you have to walk away from the problem for a while and think about it from different points of view, and about the advantages and disadvantages of possible solutions.

10. You should make a conscientious effort to evaluate the logic and credibility of what you hear. Our mind functions at some 500 words a minute, but we normally speak at 125 words a minute. In other words, we can think four times faster than we can speak. Rather than letting our minds become bored, we can take advantage of this time differential between thinking and speaking. We can attempt to anticipate the speaker's next point, attempt to identify and evaluate supporting material, and mentally summarize what the speaker has said: What has thus far been said that I can use?

Remember, listening makes the people you are listening to feel special; sometimes it enables them to solve their own problems. Perhaps they are in the process of hearing themselves think aloud on a subject for the first time. At such times, they might just want others to listen. If you refrain from injecting yourself into the conversation, you might be able to help them resolve their own internal conflicts.

As a professional, you are paid to listen. Yet studies at the University of Minnesota, confirmed by studies at Florida and Michigan State Universities, showed that people forget one-third to one-half of what they hear within eight hours.[5]

The art of listening is a skill, however, and it can be improved. You listen best when you develop a positive attitude toward listening. The first step is to become aware of the fact that listening is not a passive activity. Also, there is little correlation between intelligence and listening. You must "want" to remember.

One technique that nurses can use to improve their listening ability is to pretend that they will be quizzed later in the day about what they have heard. The health care professionals who improve their listening ability can make significant contributions to their health care teams. Only by listening to one another can we share our dreams, hopes, and fears and exchange ideas. This sharing is what makes a team—a group working together toward a common goal: improved patient care.

NOTES

1. Bill Conboy, *Working Together: Communication in a Healthy Organization* (Columbus, Ohio: Charles E. Merrill Publishing Company, 1976), p. 73.
2. Ralph G. Nichols, "Listening Is a Ten Part Skill," *Nation's Business,* July, 1957, p. 56.
3. Charles M. Kelly, "Actual Listening Behavior of Industrial Supervisors as Related to Listening Ability, General Mental Ability, Selected Personality Factors and Supervisory Effectiveness," *Small Group Communication: A Reader,* ed. Robert S. Cathcart and Larry A. Samovar (Dubuque, Iowa: William C. Brown Co., Publishers, 1970), pp. 251–259.
4. Paul T. Rankin, "Listening Ability," *Proceedings of the Ohio State Educational Conference, Ninth Annual Session* (Columbus, Ohio: Ohio State University, 1929), pp. 172–183.
5. J.H. Kramar and T.R. Lewis, "Comparison of Visual and Nonvisual Listening," *Journal of Communication* 1 (1951): 16.

SUGGESTED READINGS

Barbara, Dominick A. *The Art of Listening.* Springfield, Ill.: Charles C Thomas Publisher, 1966.

_____. *How To Make People Listen to You.* Springfield, Ill.: Charles C Thomas, Publisher, 1971.

Barker, Larry L. *Listening Behavior.* Englewood Cliffs, N.J.: Prentice Hall Inc., 1971.

Byrne, Donn P. *Listening.* New York: Longman Inc., 1975.

Duker, Sam. *Listening Bibliography.* New York: Scarecrow Press, Inc., 1964.

_____. *Listening Readings.* Metuchen, N.J.: Scarecrow Press, Inc., 1966.

Erickson, Allen G. "Can Listening Efficiency Be Improved." *Journal of Communication* 4, no. 4: 53.

Kerman, Joseph. *Listen.* New York: Worth Publishing Co., 1976.

Mills, Ernest P. *Listening: Key to Communication.* New York: Petrocelli Charter Inc., 1974.

Nichols, Ralph G. "Listening Is a Ten Part Skill." *Nation's Business,* July, 1957, pp. 56–60.

_____ and Stevens, Leonard A. *Are You Listening?* New York: McGraw-Hill Book Co., 1957.

_____ and Stevens, Leonard A. "If Only Someone Would Listen." *Journal of Communication* 8, no. 1: 8.

_____ and Stevens, Leonard A. "Listening to People." *Harvard Business Review,* September–October, 1957, pp. 85–92.

Rogers, Carl R., and Farson, Richard E. *Active Listening.* Chicago: Industrial Relations Center, University of Chicago, 1955.

Strong, Linda. "Do You Know How To Listen?" *Management Review* 44: 530–535.

Toussaint, Isabella H. "A Classified Summary of Listening, 1950–1959." *Journal of Communication* 10: 125–134.

Whyte, W.H., Jr. *Is Anybody Listening?* New York: Simon and Schuster, 1952.

Zelko, Harold P. *How To Be a Good Listener.* New York: Employee Relations, 1958.

_____. "An Outline of the Role of Listening in the Communication Process." *Journal of Communication* 4: 71.

Appendix 3-A

Suggested Activities

1. Devote a nurses' seminar or seminars to a discussion of the role and function of listening as a nursing tool.

2. If possible, bring in qualified speakers and ask them to discuss listening with special reference to how it might apply to nursing. Speakers are available at a number of universities where listening is taught as a part of communication training.

3. Get permission to record an actual conference held in a hospital. During a nursing training session, ask the nurses to listen to the tape and then discuss the role that listening played or didn't play in the conference.

4. Bring nurses from different divisions together at informal meetings where they may talk and listen to each other freely. Perhaps one day a week the lunch room could be organized so that nurses who do not ordinarily get together could be seatmates.

5. Have the nurses in your nursing class listen to a public speech, council meeting, board meeting, or other event that will be covered by a local newspaper. Then ask nurses to write a report of what they heard. The next morning compare the nurses' reports to those of the newspaper reporter, presumably a professional listener.

DELIBERATIVE LISTENING REVIEW PUZZLE

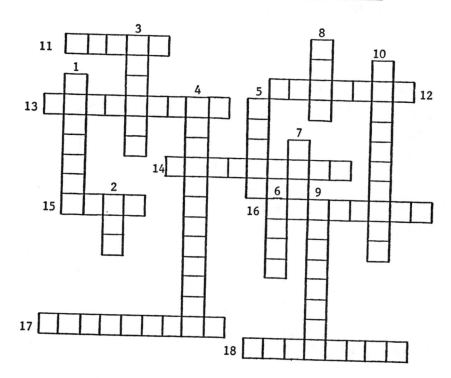

DOWN

1) Due to speed differential.
2) One type of listening response.
3) Can be reduced through good listening.
4) Can improve listening.
5) Can determine behavior.
6) A reason we may not listen.
7) Number of types of listening responses.
8) Approximate amount of time spent listening.
9) Good listening is an _____.
10) In deliberative listening we strive to _____ messages.

ACROSS

11) A type of listening response.
12) How we spend 30 percent of our communication time.
13) 68 percent of all messages.
14) Is needed to solve problems.
15) Functions at 500 words per minute.
16) The certified mail of listening.
17) 50 percent of the communicative act.
18) A synonym for attention.

(Answers are on page 50.)

DELIBERATIVE LISTENING REVIEW PUZZLE

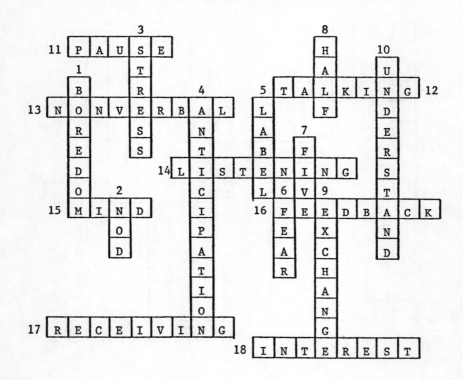

DOWN

1) Due to speed differential
2) One type of listening response.
3) Can be reduced through good listening.
4) Can improve listening.
5) Can determine behavior.
6) A reason we may not listen.
7) Number of types of listening responses.
8) Approximate amount of time spent listening.
9) Good listening is an _____.
10) In deliberative listening we strive to _____ messages.

ACROSS

11) A type of listening response.
12) How we spend 30 percent of our communication time.
13) 68 percent of all messages.
14) Is needed to solve problems.
15) Functions at 500 words per minute.
16) The certified mail of listening.
17) 50 percent of the communicative act.
18) A synonym for attention.

Chapter 4

Improved Patient Care through Active Listening

CHAPTER OBJECTIVES

The purpose of this chapter is to enable you to CHANGE your communicative behavior in a *positive* direction. After studying the material you should be able to:

Comprehend the importance of active listening.

Have an understanding of the prerequisites for active listening.

Actively listen for feelings.

Name the "attending" and "responding" functions of active listening.

Guide others toward more effective listening.

Eliminate the dysfunctional styles of responding.

Good listening habits are not the easiest of skills to develop, and that may be why many of us do it so badly. To be a good listener requires intense concentration. Research has shown that people involved in active listening show degrees of tension as they try empathically to understand what has been said.

Active listening requires the development of skills, just as deliberative listening does. It requires above all that you cannot be passive. Richard Weaver has stated: "It is an active, not a passive process. We cannot just make sure that our ears are alert or open and let the rest come naturally. Because active listening involves both emotional and intellectual inputs, it does not just happen. We have to make it happen. It takes energy and commitment."[1]

An interesting analogy between breathing habits and listening habits has been postulated by Bill Conboy:

> Doctors and biologists agree that breathing is one life process which human beings tend to handle poorly. It has been estimated that most of us could add 10 to 15 years to our life span if we practiced better breathing habits from an early age. Yet breathing is one thing we do throughout our lives. Listening habits, like breathing habits, improve only with systematic and evaluated practice. Real listening requires an expenditure of energy in obtaining and retaining the spoken discourse of others. Tests in the physiological psychology laboratory have shown that active listening demands as much energy, makes a person just as tired, as comparable efforts in speaking, reading, or writing.[2]

Active and deliberative listening requires energy plus a desire to understand. Yet the two types of listening are as different as they are similar. Charles Kelly explains that the desired result of the two types is similar—the accurate understanding of verbal communication. But this understanding is achieved in different ways:

> The deliberative listener "first" has the desire to critically analyze what the speaker has said, and "secondarily" tries to understand the speaker. . . . The active listener has the desire to understand the speaker "first" and, as a result, tries to take the appropriate action. This does not mean to suggest that the active listeners are uncritical or always in agreement with what is communicated, but rather that their

primary interest is to become fully and accurately aware of what is going on.[3]

THE IMPORTANCE OF ACTIVE LISTENING

Listening provides patients with the psychological support they need for a speedy recovery. There is a positive correlation between mental health and physical health. Patients have a tendency to recover more rapidly when they understand the procedure they are going through and are provided with the proper psychological support. This means that there must be an opportunity for patients to ask questions and talk about their apprehensions. This type of talk requires an "active" listener.

Yet, a survey conducted by *Nursing 77* indicated that 77 percent of the 10,000 nurses surveyed rated doctors as either fair or poor with respect to the psychological support they gave their patients. In such cases, the communicative (listening) therapy must be provided by the nurse.

Good active listening requires that we listen for all possible meanings—those behind the words as well as the obvious meanings. Richard Weaver suggests:

> To listen effectively we have to pay attention to facial expressions and eye contact, gestures and body movements, posture and dress, as well as the quality of the other person's voice, vocabulary, rhythm, rate, tone, and volume . . . listening with our third ear helps us to understand the whole message.[4]

This suggestion is especially applicable to the nurse-patient relationship. To be effective, the nurse must actively listen for feedback. The nurse must be able to listen to all meanings, of what has been said and in some cases of what has been left unsaid.

A nurse recently offered the following illustration: A patient did not take his medication as prescribed. When asked why, he said that he forgot. The nurse then gave him the medicine and told him not to forget again. At the prescribed time, the patient again failed to take his medication. When asked about it, he again said that he forgot. This happened repeatedly. Finally, the nurse began to question him more closely and started to listen "actively" to his verbal and nonverbal responses. Eventually the nurse determined that he had not forgotten to take his medication after all but rather was *afraid* to take it. No one had explained to him what the medication was for or how it would help him to recover. Once this situation was understood and an explanation was given, the patient promptly took his medication with no urging. In this case, the nurse was listening with the third ear, and active listening reduced unwarranted patient stress and anxiety.

Thus, even silence can be communication; when people refuse to communicate, they are sending out all kinds of messages.

Active listening is an important aspect of the nurse-patient relationship, but it is also important in relationships between neighbors, roommates, friends, parents, children, teachers, and students. Unfortunately, active listening is not highly valued in our society. It is brushed aside by many of us who were taught to listen only in the deliberative style. It should be remembered, however, that we do not listen only with our ears. We also listen with our eyes and our sense of touch; we listen by becoming aware of the feelings and emotions that arise within us because of our contact with others. We listen with our mind, our heart, and our imagination.

PREREQUISITES FOR ACTIVE LISTENING

Before the skills of active listening can be learned, certain preconditions must be met. Carl Rogers and Richard Farson believe that the good listener must meet four prerequisites in order to experience a mutually beneficial interaction:

1. The listener must *want* to listen.
2. The listener must be willing to suspend judgment; that means accepting the other person. This does not mean that the listener must approve of all of the behavior or attitudes of the other person; it means, however, that such approval or disapproval must be suspended throughout the interaction. If the other person is to deal with the problem responsibly, the good listener cannot make judgments or offer advice.
3. The listener must allow and encourage a statement of feelings by the other person. In order to solve problems successfully, such feelings must be acknowledged, accepted, and felt.
4. The listener must be aware of personal feelings during the interaction and must be prepared to integrate them into the interaction when appropriate.[5]

Rogers notes that "the major barrier to mutual interpersonal communication is our very natural tendency to judge, to evaluate, to approve or disapprove, the statement of the other person."[6] He goes on to say that "real communication occurs, when this evaluative tendency is avoided, when we listen with understanding. What does this mean? It means to see the expressed idea and attitude from the other person's point of view, to sense how it feels to him, to achieve his frame of reference in regard to the thing he is talking about."[7]

SKILLS IN ACTIVE LISTENING

Once the prerequisites of active listening are met, the listener is psychologically ready to listen. This psychological preparation is not yet enough, however, to achieve fully the promise of good listening. The achievement of empathy is important, but the listener must also communicate that empathy through "attending" and "responding." Gerard Egan has noted that "if I am to let you know that I understand you, I must first pay attention to you and listen to what you have to say about yourself."[8]

Here are some of the attending (nonverbal) and responding (verbal) behaviors by which an active listener expresses empathy.

Attending (nonverbal)	Responding (verbal)
• Facing the other person squarely	• Evaluative responses
• Adopting an open posture	• Interpretive responses
• Leaning toward the other person	• Supportive responses
• Maintaining good eye contact	• Probing responses
• Being relatively relaxed	• Understanding responses
• Reflecting attention through facial expressions	
• Attending with vocal cues	

Source: Adapted from Gerard Egan, *You and Me: The Skills of Communicating and Relating to Others.* Monterey, Cal.: Brooks–Cole Publishing Co., 1977, pp. 114–115, and David W. Johnson, *Reaching Out: Interpersonal Effectiveness and Self Actualization.* Englewood Cliffs, N.J., Prentice–Hall, Inc., p. 125.

Attending Responses

The nonverbal cues that indicate that the listener is attending are primarily physical: facing the other person squarely, adopting an open posture, leaning toward the other person, maintaining good eye contact, maintaining a relatively relaxed musculature, and reflecting attention through appropriate facial expressions.

Egan believes that your body can either emphasize the message yo.
are trying to communicate with words or it can erase the message you
are sending with words and even substitute an opposite message.[9]

Albert Mehrabian noted the following division of the communicative
process. He discovered that, of the total message, 7 percent is verbal,
38 percent is vocal, and 55 percent is facial.[10] Mehrabian's findings emphasize the importance of the 93 percent of the message that is nonverbal. He also notes that such nonverbal attending behaviors are indica-
tions of "caring," manifested in immediacy or liking.[11]

Becoming aware of the nonverbal is important to listeners for two
primary reasons. First, listeners can become sensitive to the value of
their own verbal cues in communicating to senders that listening is
taking place. Nurses can say through their attention, "We are here, we
are interested in you, we want to listen." Attending thus confirms for
the sender that listening is occurring. Second, listeners can become
sensitive to the total messages of senders through attention to the latter's nonverbal as well as verbal cues. Nurses' recognition of both the
verbal and nonverbal parts of messages will aid them in developing
understanding and empathy.

Responding Responses

Though paying attention is important, it does not always lead to accurate, empathic understanding between sender and listener. It is also
important to let other people know how you interpret their messages.

John Stewart and Gary D'Angelo call this process "perception
checking." They state: "When you are perception checking, you verbalize your interpretation or inferences about what was said or left unsaid, and you ask the other person to verify or correct your interpretation."[12]

Phrasing of Responses

Stewart and D'Angelo also suggest two categories of responses:
paraphrasing and parasupporting.[13] There are four rules of paraphrasing:

1. Say in your own words what you heard the other person saying.
2. Try to include some of what you perceive the other person to be
feeling.
3. Don't just "word swap." That is, do not merely repeat what the

sender has said. Repeating does little to let the sender know that the listener understands. Nor does it really encourage the sender to elaborate.

4. Give the other person a chance to verify your paraphrase.

Even attentive and active listeners are not always accurate in their interpretations. The purpose of perception checking is to determine whether or not the sender's message has been accurately interpreted and understood. If the listener has misinterpreted the sender, the good listener will admit it. Few senders will be fooled by a dishonest listener; but most will in fact appreciate an honest mistake, and the listener's trustworthiness will be enhanced.

The second dimension of perception checking suggested by Stewart and D'Angelo is parasupporting. Here, listeners will not only paraphrase what the senders have said but will also carry their own ideas further by providing examples or other data that tend to illustrate, clarify, or support the senders' feelings.[14]

DYSFUNCTIONAL STYLES OF RESPONDING

In the development of an appropriate response style, the listener might have the tendency to respond in dysfunctional ways. Egan offers eight examples.

1. *The cliche.* When someone discloses a personal problem, a response with a cliche, such as, "Oh, I know how you feel," can be less functional than no response at all. Egan believes cliches put distance between people.[16]

2. *The question.* A question can be helpful in probing, that is, in gaining information concerning the sender's problems. But a question can also be perceived as interrogation and place the other person on the defensive. With few exceptions, a question can be rephrased into a declarative statement. The purpose of gaining information is thus still served, but the possibility of defensiveness is avoided.

3. *Inaccuracy.* If your understanding of other people is inaccurate, those people may feel "blocked," that is, they may lose trust in your ability to understand and, as a result, stop the interaction. Perception checking can help the listener avoid inaccuracies.

4. *Feigning understanding.* It isn't always easy to understand what

a sender is trying to communicate, even if the listener "attends" well. But if the listener merely pretends to understand, the sender will sense this, and this will create a barrier. Egan says, "If you are confused, admit your confusion. . . . Such statements are signs of respect, of the fact that you think it is important to stay with the other."

5. *Parroting.* Mere repetition of what the other person says does little to establish empathy.

6. *Jumping in too quickly or letting the other person ramble.* The good listener will let the other person pace the interaction, unless that person begins to ramble. Listeners should feel free to interrupt if they have something important to say, but generally the senders should be in charge.

7. *Discrepancy in language, tone, or manner.* The use of idiosyncratic jargon or behavior by the listener is inappropriate. As far as possible, the listener should follow the cues from the sender so that the sender does not feel invaded.

8. *Longwindedness.* The listener's responses should be as succinct as possible. Comments should be to the point, but not too long. Remember, the sender is in control of the interaction.[15]

Other common mistakes in listening noted by Egan are indicated by the following kinds of responses:

- responses that imply condescension or manipulation
- unsolicited advice giving
- responses that indicate rejection or disrespect
- premature confrontation
- patronizing or placating responses
- responses that ignore what the person said
- use of inappropriate warmth or sympathy
- judgmental remarks
- defensive responses[16]

SUMMARY

Norman Metzger offers the following advice to improve our "deliberative" and "active" listening ability:

- Most of us talk too much. At times we should use judicious silence. Silence is a great way to motivate other people to speak up, to let us know what's on their minds.

- Most of us frame questions to get the answers we want to hear. We should frame our questions so that we leave the way open for whatever type of answer the other person wants to give. We should allow the other person time to finish the answer.
- Most of us set up communication in counterproductive atmospheres. If possible, we should pick a time or place that provides maximum comfort and minimum distraction. If the communication is an emotion-laden issue, we should pick a place of privacy and protect the dignity of all parties.
- Many of us let emotional filters get in the way of understanding. Be honest about your biases. When you feel strongly about a subject, be particularly careful. At such times there is a chance that you will misinterpret, misunderstand, and miscommunicate. The next time your emotions boil over, make a mental note regarding the time and place and people involved. You might be able to track down the source of your feelings and the trigger that sets you off.
- Most of us listen only for facts. We fail to see the topic from the other person's point of view. Listen for "feelings." Pay as much attention to the way you or someone else says something as to what is said. Pay attention to *all* meanings. Then check out your perceptions with these phrases: "I conclude that you approve (or disapprove) of . . ." or, "Am I right in concluding that what you are saying is . . . ."[17]

According to Metzger, listening is a multifaceted process that includes

- what you *mean* to say
- what you *actually* said
- what the other person *hears*
- what the other persons *think* they hear
- what the other person *says*
- what you *think* the other person says[18]

If I listen to you, there is a chance that you will listen to me. If I don't listen to you, there is very little chance you will listen to me. Good relationships between health care professionals and patients depend upon good listening. Only through good listening can we help one another and ultimately help ourselves.

Appendix 4-A

Suggested Activities

1. Form a group of three to five nurses and ask them to comment on the following statements that are often verbalized about the listening process. Explain, expand, and clarify what the group thinks is meant by each statement. Finally, determine the validity of each statement as a principle of good listening. Try to do bridge building; that is, relate your experience in personal communication to these statements to see if they accurately describe what you have experienced.

- Listening is inevitable when two people are together.
- The "punctuation" of interpersonal interactions affects the meaning conveyed to the listener.
- Listening ultimately defines an interpersonal relationship.
- Good listening habits are the easiest of all to develop.
- Listening attentively to others improves the ability to listen.

2. Role-play a situation in which a nurse does not listen to a doctor and show how this affects their communication.

3. Role-play a situation in which a doctor does not listen to a nurse and show how this affects their communication.

ACTIVE LISTENING REVIEW PUZZLE

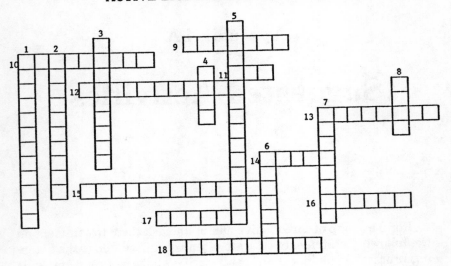

DOWN

1) A dimension of perception checking.
2) Displaying verbal listening behaviors.
3) Displaying nonverbal listening behaviors.
4) Number of paraphrasing rules.
5) A dimension of perception checking.
6) Shown by people involved in active listening.
7) The certified mail of listening.
8) The listener must_____to listen.

ACROSS

9) Requirement for active listening.
10) A dysfunctional response.
11) We should listen for ____meanings.
12) These should be checked.
13) Important in solving problems.
14) We should listen with our_____ear.
15) Should be avoided.
16) A dysfunctional response.
17) What attending behaviors indicate.
18) A poor listening attitude.

(Answers are on page 64.)

NOTES

1. Richard Weaver, *Understanding Interpersonal Communication* (Glenview, Ill.: Scott, Foresman and Co., 1978), p. 100.

2. Bill Conboy, *Working Together: Communication in a Healthy Organization* (Columbus, Ohio: Charles E. Merrill Publishing Co., 1976), pp. 73–74.

3. Charles Kelly, "Actual Listening Behavior of Industrial Supervisors as Related to Listening Ability, General Mental Ability, Selected Personality Factors and Supervisory Effectiveness," *Small Group Communication: A Reader*, ed. Robert S. Cathcart and Larry A. Samovar (Dubuque, Iowa: William C. Brown Co., Publishers, 1970), pp. 252–253.

4. Weaver, *Interpersonal Communication*, p. 99.

5. Carl R. Rogers and Richard E. Farson, "Problems in Active Listening," *Communication Probes*, B.D. Peterson, G.M. Goldhaber, and R.W. Pace, eds. (Chicago: SRA, 1974), pp. 30–34.

6. Carl R. Rogers, *On Becoming a Person* (Boston: Houghton Mifflin Co., 1961), p. 330.

7. *Ibid.*, pp. 331–332.

8. Gerard Egan, *You and Me: The Skills of Communicating and Relating to Others* (Monterey, California: Brooks-Cole Publishing Co., 1977), p. 109.

9. *Ibid.*, p. 113.

10. Albert Mehrabian, *Silent Messages* (Belmont, California: Wadsworth Publishing Co., 1971), p. 43.

11. *Ibid.*, pp. 1–23.

12. John Stewart, and Gary D'Angelo, *Together: Communicating Interpersonally* (Reading, Mass.: Addison-Wesley, 1975), p. 192.

13. *Ibid.*, p. 195.

14. *Ibid.*, p. 193.

15. Gerard Egan, *Interpersonal Living* (Monterey, California: Brooks-Cole Publishing Co., 1976), pp. 124–129.

16. *Ibid.*, p. 131.

17. Norman Metzger, *The Health Care Supervisor's Handbook* (Germantown, Maryland: Aspen Systems Corp.), pp. 60–61.

18. *Ibid.*, p. 62.

SUGGESTED READINGS

Barbara, Dominick A. "On Listening: The Role of the Ear in Psychic Life." *Today's Speech* 5, no. 1: 12–15.

Nichols, Ralph G. "Factors in Listening Comprehension." *Speech Monographs* 15: 154.

Reik, Theodor. *Listening With the Third Ear*. New York: Grove Press, 1948.

Rogers, Carl R., and Farson, Richard E. *Problems in Active Listening*. Chicago, Ill.: Industrial Relations Center, The University of Chicago, 1974.

———. *On Becoming a Person*. Boston: Houghton Mifflin Company, 1961.

Weaver, Carl H. *Human Listening: Processes and Behavior*. New York: The Bobbs-Merrill Company, Inc., 1972.

ACTIVE LISTENING REVIEW PUZZLE

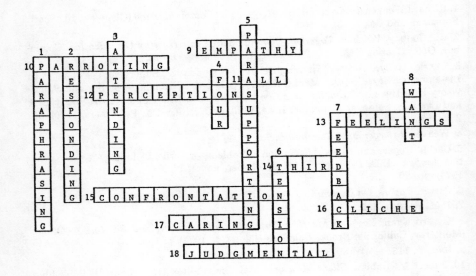

DOWN

1) A dimension of perception checking.
2) Displaying verbal listening behaviors.
3) Displaying nonverbal listening behaviors.
4) Number of paraphrasing rules.
5) A dimension of perception checking.
6) Shown by people involved in active listening.
7) The certified mail of listening.
8) The listener must_____to listen.

ACROSS

9) Requirement for active listening.
10) A dysfunctional response.
11) We should listen for ____meanings.
12) These should be checked.
13) Important in solving problems.
14) We should listen with our_____ear.
15) Should be avoided.
16) A dysfunctional response.
17) What attending behaviors indicate.
18) A poor listening attitude.

Chapter 5

The Dynamics of Nursing Leadership

CHAPTER OBJECTIVES

The purpose of this chapter is to enable you to CHANGE your communicative behavior in a *positive* direction. After studying the material you should be able to:

Compare the differences between the interactional and trait approaches of leadership.

Have an understanding of the "task" and "maintenance" functions of leadership.

Assess your knowledge of leadership.

Notice leadership potential in others.

Generate a new style of personal leadership.

Evaluate your own leadership ability.

Little can be accomplished without some predetermined plan of action. In fact, by definition, to accomplish means to meet a goal. To reach and meet goals requires leadership. Thus, to meet early twentieth century goals, most organizations were directed by autocratic or paternalistic leaders. Workers were willing to listen and respond to the boss or the expert. Now, in the latter half of the century, workers are more apt to question authority. This questioning attitude on the part of workers is commonly referred to as the psychology of job entitlement.

In the early part of the twentieth century, the problem of leadership did not seem as severe as it is today. In politics, business, and education, certain people were designated as the experts; and voters, employees, and students tended to think of the world as being divided into leaders and followers. In short, our society was much less complex than it is today.

In the last ten years, however, Los Angeles has grown by 2.5 million. In July, 1964, the population of the United States was about 192 million. The U.S. Census Bureau estimates that the population in 1980 will be between 246 and 260 million. Today, more than half of all Americans were born after World War II and are under 35 years of age.

Forty years ago, only one out of every eight Americans had gone to high school. Today, four out of five attend high school. Forty years ago, less than 4 percent of the population attended college. Now the figure is around 40 percent. These changes have stimulated new approaches to the study of leadership.

There have been more than 1,800 studies of leadership, but there is still little agreement on how to describe, identify, or evaluate it. Leadership effectiveness has many different dimensions; effective leaders must meet the interpersonal needs of the groups they lead.

Early research on leader effectiveness was centered on the leader. Gradually, however, the concept of group dynamics emerged from the social sciences with a focus primarily on members of the group rather than solely on the leader.

The new approach stemmed primarily from Kurt Lewin and his associates in the late 1930s and early 1940s. The group dynamics movement stressed the larger human element rather than merely the thinking element in group behavior. This larger emphasis provided researchers with new insights into the interactions between leader and follower.

Andrew Halpin notes that there are two main components of leadership—task and individual behavior—that appear to play significant roles in the interaction between leaders and followers.[1]

Other writers refer to the needs of group members in defining task and individual behavior. William Sattler and N. Edd. Miller believe that task-oriented leaders deal with problem-solving functions; they ask to have goals identified, ask for information, give information, evaluate information, resolve differences, and call for plans of action. The task-oriented leader is mainly interested in getting the job done, regardless of personal feelings.[2]

On the other hand, the leader oriented toward the individual shows a willingness to reveal signs of friendliness, warmth, respect, and mutual trust. Through this type of behavior, leaders can attempt to eliminate their followers' feelings of anxiety, strain, tension, embarrassment, and discomfort.[3]

It should be kept in mind that the dimensions of task and individual behavior are not mutually exclusive categories. The components of task-oriented behavior and individual-oriented behavior tend to cross-stimulate one another. Here, however, we will separate the two dimensions to have more distinct components for purposes of analysis.

THE LEADER AND THE GROUP

Richard Heslin and Dexter Dunphy prepared detailed abstracts of 450 small group studies and then analyzed those studies that dealt with group satisfaction. Their findings were that member satisfaction is high when (1) either a leader emerges who is effective in both the task and individual functions of the group, or two complementary leaders emerge with one handling the task functions and the other handling the individual functions; and (2) the designated leader or leaders are perceived by the group members to be competent.[4]

As noted earlier, the two leadership behaviors are not mutually exclusive. The nurse should remember that the dual role of leadership sometimes requires movement away from democratic, group-centered leadership toward autocratic leadership. On the other hand, the nursing leader's belief in the democratic process, in the ability of members of the group to solve their own problems, tends to pull the nursing leader back to group-centered, democratic leadership. When the need for both approaches is recognized, the leadership will be suited to the group and to the situation.

Carl Rogers notes that the extent to which leader characteristics affect a group is not clearly known. One hypothesis suggests that group members identify with their leader and in the process internalize some of their leader's characteristics of leadership. This might mean that members of a group will begin to behave toward other group members in much the same way that their leader behaves toward them. They would become more friendly and warm toward others in the group, more empathic in their relations with others, if their leader's behavior were also oriented toward this end.[5]

Hanan Selvin studied the differences between what he called "persuasive climate" and "arbitrary climate." He points to the need to establish a climate of psychological safety and refers to the dual roles of leadership and how each influences the other. He found that persuasive climates reduced tension and tended to satisfy personal needs more than arbitrary climates. He also found that a personal, non-threatening climate improved task efficiency.[6]

THE LEADERSHIP SELECTION PROCESS

Most social psychologists and experts on communication agree on certain basic characteristics of leadership. Before we proceed to establish criteria for leadership selection, see how closely you agree with the experts by taking this brief test. Decide whether each statement is more true or more false. The answers and test rationale will be given later in this chapter.

TRUE FALSE

_____ _____ 1. Leaders are born not made.

_____ _____ 2. Leadership should be a reward for loyalty or length of service.

_____ _____ 3. Only extroverts can be effective leaders.

_____ _____ 4. You can tell leaders by their neat appearances.

_____ _____ 5. The more automatic and habitual the thinking and action of leaders, the more democratic their leadership will become.

_____ _____ 6. Effective leaders often forget about a problem for a while in order to solve it.

_____ _____ 7. A leader with a deep interest in people will normally be more effective than a leader who is interested only in getting the job done.

_____ _____ 8. Leaders are best suited to select future leaders.

_____ _____ 9. In most cases, how people behaved in the past will determine their future behavior.

_____ _____ 10. Leadership effectiveness is dependent upon the situation.

The Trait Approach

The trait approach attempts to list characteristics that "good" leaders have in common. These traits might be enthusiasm, friendliness, direction, integrity, skill, intelligence, and courage. For many years, it was believed that good leaders could be identified by observing their characteristics, that certain traits set leaders apart from people who were not destined to be leaders. An examination of the studies on leadership, however, reveals the major weakness of the trait approach: seldom do the suggested lists of traits agree on the essential elements of leadership.

R.M. Stogdill surveyed over 100 studies of leadership. He discovered that less than five percent of the traits reported as effective leadership characteristics were common in four or more of the studies surveyed. He also found evidence that suggested that leaders cannot be too different from their followers and that followers must be able to identify with their leader.[7]

The Interactional Approach

The early studies on leadership that depended almost exclusively on the trait approach tended to disregard the importance of interactions between leaders and followers. More recently, however, the staff of the Ohio State Leadership Studies discovered as a result of its investigations that it is more meaningful to speak of the "leader behavior" of people rather than their leadership capacity or ability. This allows one to speak about what people do when they are leading. When leadership is thought about in this way, attention is focused on the interaction of people and the roles they play in a group situation. This approach thus appears to be more meaningful than the trait approach in selecting leaders. In the interactional approach, the leadership acts are identified, and the group interactions can be described quite reliably. In contrast, the trait approach provides little assurance that persons having certain traits—such as personality, skill, ability, or intelligence—could be depended upon to lead in all situations. The trait approach examines only the static characteristics of people; it does not describe the dynamics of leadership as a process.[8]

The interactional approach can be best summarized in the following points:

- Leadership is a product of the interaction that takes place among individuals in a group; it is not a product of the status or position of these individuals.

- Activity by an individual that tends to clarify thinking, create better understanding, or otherwise cause group action is called leader behavior or leader activity.
- The effectiveness of leader behavior is measured in terms of mutuality of goals, productivity, and the maintenance of group solidarity.

These summary points touch upon a key point of leadership. Normally we think that only designated leaders perform leadership functions. But, as indicated, any activity by an individual in a group that tends to clarify thinking, create better understanding, or otherwise cause group action is leader behavior or leader activity. Such behavior by an undesignated leader is often referred to as the dynamics of personal leadership. Every nurse has a responsibility to exhibit leader behavior when the situation warrants it. The designated leader doesn't always have all of the answers to all of the problems. At times, the individual members of a nursing team, through the dynamics of personal leadership, can help to solve problems and meet group goals.

All organizations require leadership. In most cases, people are promoted from within an organization to positions of supervision. How should these people be chosen? An important rule is that a nurse should not be chosen for a position of leadership without obtaining some feedback from that nurse's coworkers. Indeed, coworkers, the people who work with the nurse on an equal basis, have an opportunity to develop a keener insight into the nurse's behavior than the higher echelon of management. This is especially true at the level of interpersonal needs.

It follows that hospital administrators and nursing supervisors should seek feedback from a nurse's coworkers before selecting that nurse for a position of leadership. This data should play a significant role in the selection process. For example, answers to the following questions about a nurse's working conditions will indicate that nurse's future leadership behavior:

- Does the nurse attempt to see the other person's point of view? (This doesn't mean does the nurse always agree with the other person.)
- Can the nurse disagree without being disagreeable?
- Does the nurse listen to and not just hear other people? (There is a real difference between listening and hearing; listening suggests that the nurse is at least trying to understand how the

other person feels about things.)

- Is the nurse responsible? When given an assignment, does the nurse follow through?
- Can the nurse be trusted? When the nurse says something, can we believe it?
- Can I identify with the nurse in some way? Is the nurse one of us working toward a common goal?
- Does the nurse give others the opportunity to express their ideas?
- Is the nurse enthusiastic? Can the nurse transfer that enthusiasm to others?
- Does the nurse encourage coworkers and compliment them on a good job?
- Most important, is the nurse more interested in the welfare of other people and of the organization than in personal recognition?

In order to maintain effective health care practices, a hospital must select the right people for positions of supervision, and nursing team members must realize that they are dependent upon one another to get the job done. No group can succeed by working in isolation. Rather they must care about one another and work toward a common goal. This team spirit produces what may be called a group or organizational climate.

A group climate is the collective view of people within an organization regarding the nature of the environment in which they work. The climate is dependent upon both the leadership and the workers of the organization. It may initially appear that the leader plays a minor role in the establishment of a group climate. This is not the case; the leader, by focusing attention on factors of group climate, can change that climate very rapidly.

The establishment of a positive group climate that stimulates employee motivation and heightens staff morale will be determined by how the leader's "task" and "individual" behaviors are combined in the group. The leader can exhibit four possible leadership behaviors:

1. high task and high individual behavior
2. high task and low individual behavior
3. high individual and low task behavior
4. low task and low individual behavior

Research studies indicate that nurses' job satisfaction is highest when their leaders exhibit "high task" and "high individual" behavior.

The following Leadership Style Questionnaire will provide some insights into your leadership behaviors, whether those behaviors are those of a designated leader or of a member exhibiting the dynamics of personal leadership within a group. After determining your leadership profile, you will be able to compare it with a composite profile of 150 nursing supervisors representing over 100 hospitals. The composite profile was obtained by tabulating data from the Leadership Style Questionnaire gathered at the third annual *Hospital Topics* Nursing Conference held in Los Angeles in 1976.

Leadership Style Questionnaire

This is not a test with right or wrong answers. It is a questionnaire designed to describe some of your attitudes about leadership. Below are ten statements about situations. After each statement, there are three possible behaviors or actions indicated that you might take if placed in a position of leadership. Place a number 3 beside the position you would *most likely* take, a number 2 beside the position you would *next likely* take, and a number 1 beside the position you would *least likely* take.

For each question you should have three answers: a 3 for your preferred behavior or action, a 2 for your second choice, and a 1 for your least likely choice.

---

1. *In Leading a Meeting It Is Important To:*
   - keep the focus on the agenda at hand . . . . (1)____
   - focus on each individual's feelings and help people express their emotional reactions to the issue . . . . (2)____
   - focus on the differing perceptions people have and how they deal with each other . . . . (3)____
2. *A Primary Objective of a Leader Is:*
   - to maintain an organizational climate in which learning and accomplishment can take place . . . . . . (4)____
   - to maintain the efficient operation of the organization . . . . (5)____
   - to help members of the organization find themselves and be more aware of who they are . . . . (6)____

3. *When Strong Disagreement Occurs Between a Leader
and a Group Member About Work To Be Done, the
Leader Should:*
- listen to the person and try to discover how
that person might have misunderstood the task .... (7)____
- try to get other people to express their views
in order to involve them in the issues .... (8)____
- support the group member for raising the
question or disagreement .... (9)____

4. *In Evaluating a Group Member's Performance,
the Leader Should:*
- involve the entire group in setting goals
and in evaluating one another's performance ...... (10)____
- try to make an objective assessment of each
person's accomplishments and effectiveness ..... (11)____
- allow individual members to be involved in
determining their own goals and performance
standards .... (12)____

5. *When Two Group Members Get into an Argument, It
Is Best To:*
- help them deal with their feelings as a means
of resolving the argument .... (13)____
- encourage other members to respond to the
argument and to try to help resolve it .... (14)____
- allow some time for expression of both sides,
but keep in focus the relevant subject matter
and the task at hand .... (15)____

6. *The Best Way To Motivate Group Members Who Are
Not Performing Up to the Best of Their Ability
Is To:*
- point out to them the importance of the
job to be done and their role in it .... (16)____
- try to get to know them better so you can
understand why they are not realizing their
potential .... (17)____
- show them how their lack of motivation is affecting other people .... (18)____

7. *The Most Important Element in Judging Group
   Members' Performance Is:*
   - their technical skill and ability .... (19)____
   - how they get along with their peers and how
     they help others learn and get the work done ...... (20)____
   - their success in meeting the goals they set
     for themselves .... (21)____

8. *In Dealing with Minority Group Issues,
   A Leader Should:*
   - deal with such issues as they threaten to
     disturb the atmosphere of the work group .... (22)____
   - be sure that all group members understand
     the history of racial and ethnic minorities in
     the community and country .... (23)____
   - help group members to achieve an under-
     standing of their own attitudes toward
     people of other races and cultures .... (24)____

9. *A Leader's Goal Should Be To:*
   - make sure that all group members have a
     solid foundation of knowledge and skills that
     will help them become productive and effective
     people .... (25)____
   - help people to learn to work effectively in
     groups, to use the resources of the group, and
     to understand their relationships with one
     another as people .... (26)____
   - help group members become responsible for
     their own education and effectiveness........... (27)____

10. *The Trouble with Leadership Responsibilities Is That:*
    - they make it very difficult to cover adequately
      all the details that must be attended to .... (28)____
    - they keep a leader from really getting to know
      group members as individuals .... (29)____
    - they make it difficult for the leader to keep in
      touch with the climate and pulse of the group ..... (30)____

SCORING

Note that, in scoring the questionnaire, the scoring columns are not in the usual sequential order.

SCORING COLUMNS

INSTRUCTIONS	TASK	INDIVIDUAL	CLIMATE
1. Transfer your answers from	(1)____	(2)____	(3)____
the Leadership Style Ques-	(5)____	(6)____	(4)____
tionnaire to the scoring col-	(7)____	(9)____	(8)____
umns at right, placing a 1,	(11)____	(12)____	(10)____
2, or 3 beside each ques-	(15)____	(13)____	(14)____
tion number.	(16)____	(17)____	(18)____
2. Add up your totals for each	(19)____	(21)____	(20)____
column. The three totals	(23)____	(24)____	(22)____
combined should equal	(25)____	(27)____	(26)____
60.	(28)____	(29)____	(30)____
3. Mark your score for	TOTAL____	TOTAL____	TOTAL____

3. Mark your score for each dimension on the bar graph below. Blacken in the bar from the left to your score on each dimension.

|←——low——→|←——high——→|

TASK

INDIVIDUAL

CLIMATE

0   5   10   15   20   25   30

4. The completed bars represent your leadership profile at this moment in time.

HOW TO INTERPRET YOUR LEADERSHIP PROFILE

1. Three bars of similar length (within variations of two or three points) indicate that you try to balance your concerns for task, feelings, and climate.

2. The longest bar tends to symbolize your characteristic leadership style in most situations. This style is probably functional for you most of the time, but it may be overused.

3. The shortest bar indicates an area you may tend to overlook. You might improve the situation by placing more emphasis on the leadership style represented by that bar.

4. You will improve your leadership the fastest by attending to issues symbolized by the shorter bars.

NURSING SUPERVISORS
COMPOSITE LEADERSHIP STYLE PROFILE

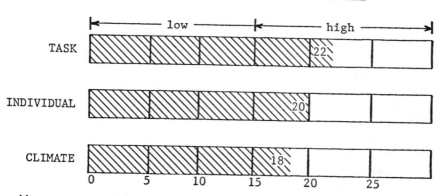

You may now wish to compare your leadership profile with the composite profile obtained at the third annual *Hospital Topics* Nursing Conference held in Los Angeles, in 1976.

Earlier in this chapter you were asked to take a test on your knowledge of leadership. The answers and their rationale are presented below:

1. Leaders are born not made. FALSE. Research indicates that environmental factors and proper training play a significant role in the development of leadership abilities.

2. Leadership should be a reward for loyalty or length of service. FALSE. Only the most sincere, energetic, and capable individuals who have a desire to serve should be appointed to positions of leadership. Loyalty is important, but leadership requires more than just loyalty.

3. Only extroverts can be effective leaders. FALSE. To be a leader, one must have visibility. However, many reserved and quiet people exhibit tremendous leadership ability when given the opportunity to express themselves.

4. You can tell leaders by their neat appearances. FALSE. We should be more interested in what leaders do when they are leading. Their ideas, their attitudes, their ability to motivate others are more important than the first impressions they make.

5. The more automatic and habitual the thinking and action of leaders, the more democratic their leadership will become. FALSE. Automatic and habitual reactions portray highly directive, autocratic leadership.

6. Effective leaders often forget about a problem for a while in order to solve it. TRUE. Sometimes it is best to walk away from a problem for a while. This gives the leader the opportunity to look at the problem and examine it from many different points of view.

7. A leader with a deep interest in people will normally be more effective than a leader who is interested only in getting the job done. TRUE. Leadership does depend upon the situation, but a leader with a deep interest in people will be better able to get the job done time and time again. A leader interested only in the job may get that particular job done, but what about the next job?

8. Leaders are best suited to select future leaders. FALSE. Research has shown that leaders should be selected by how well they work and interact with the people they are to lead. Appointed leaders may work well with the person who appointed them, but how do they work with the people they are to lead? A leader must have followers, for without followers there is no need for a leader.

9. In most cases, how people behaved in the past will determine their future behavior. TRUE. Remember, the statement applies to "most cases" and does not mean to suggest that a person cannot ever change. On the other hand, if a person has been a hard worker and reliable and conscientious over a long period of time, the chances that that person will stay that way are pretty good.

10. Leadership effectiveness is dependent upon the situation. TRUE. A leader cannot always respond to everyone in the same

way. The behavior of leaders will be determined to a large extent by the attitudes and training of their followers.

If you scored nine or ten of the statements correctly, you are going in the right direction and have an excellent awareness of the meaning of leadership. If you scored seven or eight correctly, you are at times uncertain about the way to go, and you have some misconceptions about leadership that may limit your ability to lead effectively. If you scored less than seven correctly, you need to work on your leadership awareness and capabilities.

Appendix 5-A

Suggested Activities

1. Interview several persons who, in your opinion, are successful leaders in your health care organization and in your community. Ask them to express their philosophy of leadership. After the interviews, compare their philosophies and attempt to determine if there are any common characteristics of leadership. Then interview several followers of the leaders you interviewed and ask them why they consider their leaders to be successful or unsuccessful. After these interviews, compare the comments and attempt to determine if there are any common characteristics that tend to make leaders successful or unsuccessful.

2. The following are often considered to be primary characteristics of leadership:

   a. All leaders have followers.
   b. Leaders often seek leadership roles so forcefully that they drive their followers away.
   c. Leaders are always "good" guys.
   d. Effective leaders are extroverts.
   e. Leaders should not get too close to their followers.

Form a small group of three to five nurses and ask them to comment on at least three of the above statements. Explain, expand, and clarify what is meant by each statement. Finally, determine the validity of each statement as a principle of "good" leadership. Try to do bridge building, that is, the nurses should relate their personal experiences to the statements to see if they accurately describe what they have experienced.

LEADERSHIP REVIEW PUZZLE

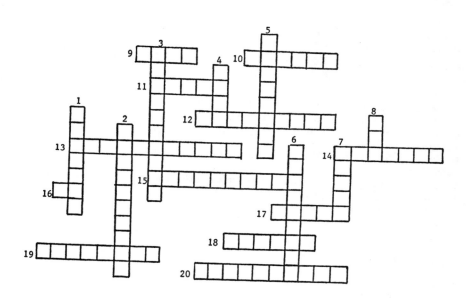

DOWN

1) A collective group view.
2) A necessary element in order to achieve a group goal.
3) Highly directive leadership.
4) Initials of behaviors for ideal leadership.
5) Needed to implement change in existing policies.
6) Leaders must have these.
7) They accurately perceive interpersonal needs.
8) The number of major leadership components.

ACROSS

9) Behavior that emphasizes getting the job done.
10) Those whom a leader leads.
11) An approach used to pick leaders.
12) A variable that leadership is dependent upon.
13) What a leader should encourage in a group.
14) A way to conceive of the role of leadership.
15) Behavior that emphasizes human considerations.
16) Initials of behavior indicating little job interest.
17) Should be determined by the leader and group together.
18) Effective leaders do this often.
19) Group energy.
20) An "individual" kind of behavior.

(Answers are on page 84.)

NOTES

1. Andrew Halpin, "Evaluation Through the Study of the Leader's Behavior," *Perspectives on the Group Process,* ed. C. Kemp (Boston: Houghton-Mifflin Professional Publishers, 1964), pp. 264–265.
2. William Sattler and N. Edd. Miller, *Discussion and Conference* (Englewood Cliffs, N.J.: Prentice-Hall Inc., 1968), pp. 213–214.
3. *Ibid.,* pp. 213–214.
4. Richard Heslin and Dexter Dunphy, "Three Dimensions of Member Satisfaction in Small Groups," *Human Relations* 17 (1964): 99–112.
5. Carl Rogers, *Client Centered Therapy* (Boston: Houghton-Mifflin Professional Publishers, 1951), pp. 348–349.
6. Hanan C. Selvin, *The Effects of Leadership* (Glencoe, Ill.: Free Press of Glencoe, 1960), p. 45.
7. R.M. Stogdill, "Personal Factors Associated with Leadership: A Survey of the Literature," *Journal of Psychology* 25 (1948): 64.
8. William Alexander, *Leadership for Improving Instruction* (Washington, D.C.: Association for Supervision and Curriculum Development, 1960), p. 109.

SUGGESTED READINGS

Bass, Bernard. *Leadership Psychology and Organizational Behavior.* New York: Harper & Row, 1960.

Bennett, Addison. "New Thinking Required for Development of Management Effectiveness." *Hospitals* 50: 67–70.

Fiedler, Fred E., and Chemers, Martin. *Leadership and Effective Management.* Glenview, Ill.: Scott, Foresman and Co., 1974.

Gordon, Thomas. *Leadership Effectiveness Training.* New York: Wyden Books, 1977.

Kuriloff, Arthur H. "An Experiment in Management: Putting Theory Y to the Test." *Personnel* 40: 8–17.

Liberman, Robert P.; King, Larry W.; DeRisi, William J.; and McCann, Michael. *Personal Effectiveness: Guiding People to Assert Themselves and Improve Their Social Skills.* Champaign, Ill.: Research Press, 1975.

McMurray, Robert M. "Are You the Kind of Boss People Want to Work For?" *Business Management* 28: 59–60.

Myers, M. Scott. *Every Employee a Manager: More Meaningful Work Through Job Enrichment.* New York: McGraw-Hill Book Co., 1970.

Nealy, S.M., and Blood, M.R. "Leadership Performance of Nursing Supervisors at Two Organizational Levels." *Journal of Applied Psychology* 52: 120–129.

———, and Owen, T.M. "A Multitrait-Multimethod Analysis of Predictors and Criteria of Nursing Performance." *Organizational Behavior and Human Performance* 5: 348–365.

Nuckolls, Katherine B. "Who Decides What a Nurse Can Do?" *Nursing Outlook* 22: 626–631.

Peter, Lawrence. *The Peter Principle.* New York: Morrow, 1969.

———. *The Peter Prescription.* New York: Morrow, 1972.

Phelps, Stanley, and Austin, Nancy. *The Assertive Woman.* San Luis Obispo, Calif.: Impact Press, 1975.

Preston, M., and Heinz, R. "Effects of Participatory Versus Supervisory Leadership on Group Judgment." *Journal of Abnormal and Social Psychology* 44: 345-355.

Stevens, Barbara J. *The Nurse as Executive.* Wakefield, Mass.: Contemporary Publishing, 1975.

Stogdill, R. "Personal Factors Associated with Leadership: A Survey of the Literature." *Journal of Psychology* 25: 35-71.

Townsend, Robert. *Up the Organization.* New York: Alfred A. Knopf Inc., 1970.

LEADERSHIP REVIEW PUZZLE

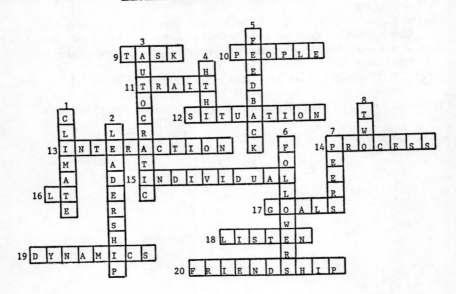

DOWN

1) A collective group view.
2) A necessary element in order to achieve a group goal.
3) Highly directive leadership.
4) Initials of behaviors for ideal leadership.
5) Needed to implement change in existing policies.
6) Leaders must have these.
7) They accurately perceive interpersonal needs.
8) The number of major leadership components.

ACROSS

9) Behavior that emphasizes getting the job done.
10) Those whom a leader leads.
11) An approach used to pick leaders.
12) A variable that leadership is dependent upon.
13) What a leader should encourage in a group.
14) A way to conceive of the role of leadership.
15) Behavior that emphasizes human considerations.
16) Initials of behavior indicating little job interest.
17) Should be determined by the leader and group together.
18) Effective leaders do this often.
19) Group energy.
20) An "individual" kind of behavior.

Chapter 6

The Nurse's Use of Nonverbal Communication

CHAPTER OBJECTIVES

The purpose of this chapter is to enable you to CHANGE your communicative behavior in a *positive* direction. After studying the material you should be able to:

Comprehend the fact that you are constantly sending nonverbal messages.

Have an understanding of the nonverbal variables that affect relationships.

Assess the nonverbal messages of your colleagues and patients.

Note that nonverbal behavior is culturally derived.

Gain an ability to recognize and be able to respond to nonverbal feedback.

Examine nonverbal meaning.

As a nurse, how often have you heard a coworker or patient say, "Seeing is believing. Did you see the way he acted when I said . . .?" Or, "I can tell by the look on her face." Or "I knew he would act that way!" All of these statements reflect a belief that the nonverbal message expresses the truth more than the verbal message. Sometimes we miss the nonverbal messages that are sent to us, indicating "I don't understand;" "Leave me alone;" "Help me, I'm depressed;" or "I think I understand, but tell me more."

NONVERBAL FEEDBACK

Nonverbal feedback provides nurses with a tool to discriminate more accurately between what is being said verbally and what is "really" being said nonverbally. The insight gained from such feedback enables nurses to anticipate problems and to help people to the extent that they are able to recognize and respond to the nonverbal feedback.

Abne Eisenberg and Ralph Smith tell us that the real distinction between verbal and nonverbal communication is that verbal behavior is organized by a language system, whereas nonverbal behavior is not.[1]

Another important distinction is that, unlike nonverbal behavior, verbal expressions are self-reflexive; that is, language can be used to talk about language. In short, you can talk about language by using language, but you can't analyze a wave of the hand with a wave of the hand.[2]

WE ARE ALWAYS COMMUNICATING

Everyone sends two messages at the same time. People send one message verbally and the other message nonverbally, through facial expressions, eye contact, tone of voice or paralanguage, touching, bodily action, and the use of space. When the nonverbal messages are congruent and tend to support the verbal message, we have clear meaningful communication. However, when the nonverbal message appears to be in conflict with the verbal message, we have unclear and faulty communication.

Ray Birdwhistell noted in the Paul Swain Lecture Series at North Carolina State University that

> Body language and spoken language are dependent on each other. Spoken language by itself will not give us the

full meaning of what a person is saying. Body language alone will not give us the total meaning. If we listen to only the words the person is saying, we may get as much distortion as if we only listen to the body language. However, 55 percent of the social meaning in a conversation is transmitted nonverbally, and in its proper context even silence is communication.[3]

Patients may choose to stop talking, but they do not cease to communicate. Have you ever tried to talk to patients, but they won't talk to you? How do you feel about administering medication to a patient who won't communicate? You may not realize it, but such a patient is sending you all kinds of nonverbal messages. To quote Sigmund Freud: "No mortal can keep a secret. If his lips are silent he chatters with his finger tips; betrayal oozes out of him at every pore."[4]

Gail and Michelle Myers tell us that it is impossible not to communicate. The nature of human communication is such that it is unavoidable. We can refrain from communication with words, but we cannot avoid nonverbal communication, . . . we cannot stop exhibiting bodily actions and facial expressions.[5]

THE IMPACT OF NONVERBAL MESSAGES

Nonverbal behaviors normally have a high degree of credibility in the mind of the beholder. Most nurse recruiters tend to agree. "I make up my mind fast, in less than five minutes," stated one nurse recruiter; "Sometimes I take a second look, but seldom change my mind." The same sentiment was expressed at a recent workshop of the North Carolina Directors of Hospital Personnel Services. One director said, "I look for nonverbal cues to support what is being said. My first impression is based on appearance, facial expression, eye contact, and gestures. A sloppy applicant is at a disadvantage especially at hospitals that don't have dress codes. I believe that clothing is an extension of self and the nonverbal behavior of applicants truly expresses their personality and attitude."

E.C. Webster found that interviewers formed an initial impression of an applicant within the first four or five minutes of the interview and then tended to search for additional information that supported and substantiated their initial impressions.[6]

Mehrabian found in the situations he examined that only 7 percent of the total impact of communication was verbal. Another 38 percent of the impact was based on how the words were said; and the remaining 55 percent was based on facial expressions, gestures, and bodily action.[7]

FORMS OF NONVERBAL COMMUNICATION

Facial Expressions

More than 100 years ago, Charles Darwin wrote *The Expression of Emotions in Man and Animals*, the product of a century-old pursuit and one of the first works on facial expression.[8] Darwin theorized that facial expressions are instinctive and not learned behavior. However, today most anthropologists believe that facial expressions are a result of natural reactions in the muscles and nerves of the face and of cultural conditioning that governs the expression of emotion.

There are six basic facial expressions: disgust, surprise, happiness, anger, sadness, and fear. Several of these expressions can be exhibited at the same time. A nurse can simultaneously exhibit surprise and disgust or surprise and happiness.

The problem of interpretation is compounded when the verbal message seems to be in conflict with the facial expression. Most nonverbal theorists agree that if the meaning of the facial expression is clear and the verbal context in which it occurs is not, the face will be the most reliable source.

P. Ekman, W.V. Friesen, and P. Ellsworth conducted an indepth analysis of all the important studies of facial expression and concluded: "Contrary to the impressions conveyed in previous reviews of the literature that the evidence in the field is confusing and contradictory, our reanalysis showed consistent evidence of accurate judgment of emotion from facial behavior."[9]

In the American culture, facial expressions play an important role in social communications between people. Facial expressions can convey true feelings and be useful communicative tools. Unfortunately, however, the general rule regarding facial expressions in America seems at times to parallel that of the ancient Greek Stoics, in that we are taught from childhood to avoid excessive expressive behavior, facial or otherwise. We are taught to show neutrality when we are angry, especially in a public place. If we are unhappy, we are urged to show only the slightest hint of sadness in our demeanor. In our culture and in many others, false facial gestures are masks behind which we hide.

Eye Contact

A look is more than just seeing. Meaning is constantly being conveyed in numerous visual ways—through the stern look of a nursing supervisor, the loving look of a patient's relative, or the caring look of a nurse. Eye contact is a highly personalized form of nonverbal communication.

As early as 1921, G. Simmel reported:

> The union and interaction of individuals is based upon mutual glances. This mutual glance between persons, in distinction from the simple sight or observation of the other, signifies a unique union between them. By the glance which reveals the other, one discloses himself. . . . The eye cannot take unless at the same time it gives.[10]

Eye contact tells us how we are doing and the kind of relationship we have with another person. We tend to look at things we like and to look away from things we dislike. Nurses who are working for the first time in paraplegic or cancer wards often have tremendous difficulty maintaining eye contact with their patients.

Michael Argyle and Janet Dean discovered that a speaker's eye contact occurs at the end of phrases and sentences but does not occur during long statements. When two people like one another, they establish eye contact more often and for a longer duration than when there is tension in the relationship.[11]

Paralanguage

It has often been said by college debaters that it's not what you say that counts, but how you say it. The tone of the voice conveys different types of meaning. Our telephone conversations, for example, rely heavily on paralanguage. The inflection in the voice, the pauses, and the rate of speech can convey anger, happiness, boredom, interest, love, hate, or frustration. Telephone conversations do not allow us the luxury of seeing gestures, facial expressions, or bodily action.

During interpersonal communication, we rely heavily on paralanguage in order to determine the genuineness of the message. Myers and Myers cite the following examples of verbal statements and what they might really mean in paralanguage:

- Verbal: "I'll be happy to do it."
  Paralanguage: "I'll do it, but it will be the last time."

- Verbal: "You always make me do what you want."
  Paralanguage: "All right you win."
- Verbal: "Don't worry I'll take care of it."
  Paralanguage: "You're so dumb I better take care of it."[12]

Touching

Some everyday verbal expressions point up the importance of touching in our daily lives: Keep in touch. He's a little touched. That really touched me. Don't be so touchy. That was a touching story. Nonverbal communication often creates a kind of intimacy seldom achieved by words alone.

In patient care, for example, nonverbal messages sent through touch often become an important way of communicating. Though eye contact is highly personalized, touching is the most intimate means of communicating through the senses. D.C. Aguilera, for example, found that touch behavior by nurses increased verbal output by patients and improved the patients' attitudes toward the nurses.[13]

The nurse should also be aware, however, that touching is potentially the most threatening type of behavior because it can degenerate into object-like control (manipulation) of another person. Touch is the most familiar of our senses, and familiarity can breed contempt when a patient feels reduced to an object. Conversely, when tactual contacts reflect "tender loving care," the patient feels comfort, confidence, acceptance, and encouragement—and responds accordingly.

Bodily Action

To a large extent, a person's social identity and self-image are created by their bodily actions. Abne Eisenberg and Ralph Smith state that "each person's psychic well being depends upon manipulating the image which he presents to others. That is, the individual's definition of himself is shaped and sustained by the reaction of other people to him. If the individual cannot elicit predictable reactions to his self presentation, then he cannot maintain a stable and consistent image of himself."[14]

Nonverbal cues, such as body position and movements of the head, express the attitudes that we have, both positive and negative, and also reflect status relationships. Mehrabian believes that movements of the limbs and head indicate not only one's attitude toward a specific set of circumstances but also how dominant and how anxious one generally tends to be in social situations.[15]

A nurse's bodily actions may be cues to let other people know that it is their turn to speak. Conversely, nurses may send cues to others indicating that they would like to comment on what has just been said. In either case, nurses, like everybody else, are constantly sending messages with their bodies.

The Use of Space

At some time or other, almost all of us have had bosses who sat and chatted with us on an office couch—until, that is, the subject turned to money or promotion, at which point they usually moved behind their desks and left us sitting alone on the couch. In this example, space can be seen to be highly personalized; all of us carry our personal space and status around with us as we stake out our territory within the limits of our influence.

Edward Hall believes that our use of space is communicative. How far people stand or sit from one another indicates how well they know one another and the purpose of their communication. Individuals send messages by placing themselves in certain spatial relationships with one another.[16]

This type of nonverbal behavior, called "proxemics," involves the relationships between the communicator's body and other people or objects in the environment. The next time you walk into a physician's or hospital administrator's office, look around to see what the room tells you. Could you walk directly into the room or did you have to gain access through a secretary?

A.G. White reported on an experiment conducted in a physician's office. He found that a desk may significantly alter a patient's at-ease state. With the desk separating the patient and doctor, only 10 percent of the patients were perceived to be at ease. When the desk was removed, the at-ease state of the patient rose to 55 percent.[17]

Distance and space tell nurses things about their working relationships. When we like people, we stand rather close to them and at times touch them. In fact, try walking down a hospital corridor with someone you like without bumping shoulders. It's almost impossible. On the other hand, if you don't like someone, it is very easy to keep a proper distance and not bump shoulders.

A personnel director at a North Carolina hospital carried out an interesting experiment. He wrote on a piece of paper the names of the people he worked with and felt close to. On the same paper he also wrote down the names of the people he worked with but didn't feel close to. Next he placed a chair by the door to his office, another chair in front of his desk, a third chair on the side of his desk, and a fourth one next to his own chair behind his desk. When people entered his office, he did not direct them to any specific chair. But after they left he wrote down where they had sat. As you might guess, he found that those he felt closest to in his working relationships sat closest to him behind his desk; indeed some even sat in his own chair.

Juluis Fast describes a set of experiments conducted by Robert Sommer, professor of psychology at the University of California:

> Dr. Sommer entered a hospital wearing a white doctor's coat, he then systematically invaded the patients' privacy, sitting next to them on benches, and entering their wards and day rooms. These intrusions, he reported, invariably bothered the patients and drove them from their special chairs or areas. The patients reacted to Dr. Sommer's physical intrusion by becoming uneasy and restless and finally by removing themselves from the area.[18]

Because personal space is invisible, people will tend to flee rather than fight if an intrusion is made into their space. Personal space can be thought of as a "plastic bubble" that surrounds the individual. When people meet, they position their bodies in such a way as to keep the walls of the bubbles intact. If one person pushes too close to another, the bubbles bounce apart.[19]

People, regardless of race or background, choose their spatial "bubbles" in the light of their own values, mores, and cultures. When other people invade their personally created private zones, they become uncomfortable, aggressive, and sometimes even hostile.

According to Hall, there are three major interpersonal distances that govern our interpersonal relationships: (1) an intimate distance from 3 to 20 inches, (2) a social distance from 20 inches to 5 feet, and (3) a public distance from 5 feet to 100 feet.[20]

CULTURAL DIFFERENCES

In dealing with various ethnic groups it is important for nurses to remember that the nonverbal behaviors of one group will not necessarily be the same as those of another group. Yet when nonverbal feedback is placed in its proper context, misinterpretations and misunderstandings between groups can be reduced.

As pointed out earlier by Hall, two to three feet from another person is a comfortable distance for most Americans for purposes of social conversation. In Brazil, Mexico, France, and most Arab countries, however, a comfortable distance for social conversation is somewhat shorter than two feet. Thus, in conversation the American is constantly moving back while a person from one of these other cultures is constantly moving forward.[21]

Here are some other differences in the behavior patterns of various cultural groups.

The Cultural Differences of Various Groups

Behavior Expressed	Behavior Pattern	Culture Group
Affection	Smelling heads	Mongols
	Rubbing noses	Eskimos
	Embracing or kissing	Eur-Americans
Approval	Smacking lips	Indians (N.A.)
	Back slapping	Eur-Americans
Assent	Elevating head	New Zealanders
	Nodding	Eur-Americans
Disrespect	Turning back and lifting skirt	French
	Snapping fingers under nose of opponents	Mediterraneans
Humility	Joining hands over head and bowing	Chinese
	Dropping arms, sighing	Europeans
	Bending body downward	Samoans
	Prostration, face down	Polynesians
Salutation	Clapping hands	Loangoan People
	Yielding up one's clothes	Assyrians
	Waving of the hand	Eur-Americans

Source: George Brown, from an unpublished graduate paper (University of Denver, Denver, 1971).

We can see from this chart that nonverbal communicative behavior must be interpreted in its proper social context. These behaviors are culturally derived and thus must be learned by nurses if they are to enjoy their maximum capacity to influence or adjust to various cultural environments.

Birdwhistell reinforces the point that there are no universal words, no sound complexes, that carry the same meaning the world over. There are no body actions, facial expressions, or gestures that provoke identical reactions in all countries.[22]

SUMMARY

More could be said about body language for didactic purposes. The core problem, however, may be that, on the one hand, we are still struggling to conceptualize the key communication variable, information, while, on the other hand, we have too little knowledge of alternative ways of interpreting the various code systems available to people. The art of nonverbal communication may be something like the statue of Venus de Milo; while interesting to look at, it still lacks the necessary hands to be an effective science. Perhaps the best way to learn the process of effective communication, verbal and nonverbal, is through the painful, difficult process that only experience can provide.

Appendix 6-A

Suggested Activities

PURPOSES

- To develop new ways of expressing one's feelings nonverbally.
- To express genuine feelings through nonverbal expression.
- To become more aware of one's nonverbal environment and the nonverbal cues one sends almost unconsciously.

DYADIC NONVERBAL EXERCISES

1. **Silent walk.** Make a silent walk across a college campus or through your hospital, taking mental notes of the various types of nonverbal communication. Note the physical characteristics (human and nonhuman), the bodily action of people, their use of touch and space. Share your observations verbally and nonverbally with another nurse.

2. **Reflecting cultural behaviors.** Express to another nurse the nonverbal behavior of a little known culture group. Then ask the nurse to guess what is being communicated.

3. **Distance.** Experiment with the comfort level of individuals by varying distances between them while sharing information that is intimate, social, and public.

4. **Trust walk.** Select a nurse to be blindfolded and to be led by a partner through and over things. Reverse the roles and repeat.

5. **Feeling objects.** Ask a blindfolded nurse to feel various medical instruments, equipment, and machines and then to name or describe the object.

6. **Invading one's territory.** Stand closer to someone than you normally would without calling attention to the fact that you are doing so. Have another nurse observe your and the other person's behaviors.

7. **Space at the dinner table.** At lunch or dinner, slowly edge your silverware, plate, and water glass past the midpoint of the table without calling attention to what you are doing. Watch as your dinner partner slowly attempts to move the objects back to your side.

SMALL GROUP NONVERBAL EXERCISES

1. **Trust roll.** Ask a group of nurses (five is an ideal number) to stand in a tight circle. Ask one of the nurses to volunteer to stand in the middle of the circle, and then, with closed eyes, to fall backward and be caught and rolled around inside the circle or thrown from side to side.

2. **Lineup.** Ask several nurses to position themselves in a line in accordance with their estimated influence in the group. Continue the exercise until the final line is satisfactory to all.

3. **Expressing emotions.** Have each nurse in the group express an emotion in turn. Have the others guess which emotion is being expressed.

MULTIGROUP NONVERBAL EXERCISES

1. **Eye contact chain.** Arrange a group of nurses in two lines, facing each other about a yard apart. Ask those at the two ends to hold hands, thus forming two linked lines similar to a bicycle chain. Instruct each person to look in the eyes of the person opposite. When everyone in the group has done so, ask each person to take one step to the right and look the new opposite person in the eyes. Continue until everybody returns to their original positions.

2. **Circles.** Ask a group of nurses to hold hands in a large circle. Now make the circle larger until it almost breaks. Then decrease the size of the circle and make it as small as possible by crowding in very close.

3. Nonverbal charades. Divide a class into six groups, with five to seven members in each group. Designate three of the groups letter teams (A, B, C) and the other three number teams (1, 2, 3). Match Team A versus Team 1, Team B versus Team 2, and Team C versus Team 3. Each team must select a timekeeper. Complete the exercise in accordance with the following rules:

- Each team selects titles within a general topic area, for example, the titles to movies, books, plays, or the names of athletic teams. Each team writes its titles or names on 3-by-5 cards and folds the cards in half.
- A member of a letter team begins the game by selecting a card from a member of a number team. The letter team silently reads the selected card and then attempts to communicate the title or name nonverbally to other members of the letter team.
- Members of the letter team may verbally ask questions and make guesses, but the member with the card can respond only nonverbally. The timekeeper from the number team times the charade and tells the groups when the three-minute time limit has elapsed.
- If the letter team guesses the title before the time is up, it receives one point. If it does not guess the title, the number team gets the point. The team with the highest score after thirty minutes wins.
- The exercise continues with letter and number teams alternating. Each team member should have an opportunity to communicate nonverbally a title or name. The titles and names must be in English and should be familiar.

NONVERBAL REVIEW PUZZLE

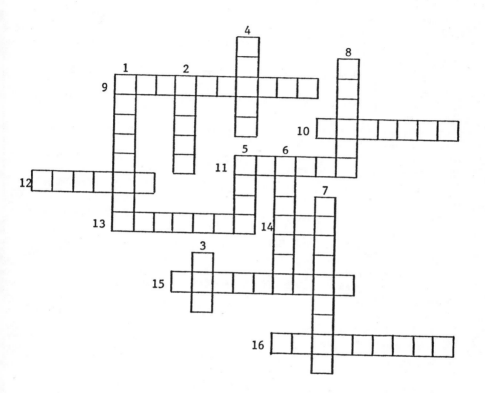

DOWN

1) An extension of self.
2) Most intimate of senses.
3) What you see is what you _____
4) One's territory.
5) Number of minutes it takes to form a first impression.
6) Nonverbal interpretation depends upon this.
7) Harmonious verbal and nonverbal messages.
8) A kind of distance, from 20 inches to five feet.

ACROSS

9) How nonverbal messages are learned.
10) A form of communication.
11) Expressions regarded as reliable indicators.
12) A kind of distance, from 5 to 100 feet.
13) A bodily action.
14) Number of basic types of messages sent at the same time.
15) We defend this.
16) The silent language.

(Answers are on page 102.)

NOTES

1. Abne Eisenberg and Ralph Smith, *Nonverbal Communication* (New York: The Bobbs-Merrill Co., 1971), p. 20.

2. Joseph DeVito, *Psychology of Speech and Language* (New York: Random House Inc., 1970), p. 8.

3. Ray Birdwhistell, *Paul Swain Lecture Series* (Raleigh, N.C.: North Carolina State University, 1974).

4. William Brooks, *Speech Communication* (Dubuque, Iowa: William C. Brown, 1974), p. 176.

5. Gail Myers and Michelle Myers, *The Dynamics of Human Communication* (New York: McGraw-Hill Book Co., 1973), p. 179.

6. Fred Fiedler and Martin Chemers, *Leadership and Effective Management* (Glenview, Ill.: Scott, Foresman and Co., 1974), p. 21.

7. Albert Mehrabian, "Communication Without Words," *Psychology Today* 2 (1968): 53.

8. Charles Darwin, *The Expression of Emotions in Man and Animals* (Chicago: University of Chicago Press, 1965).

9. P. Ekman, W.V. Friesen and P. Ellsworth, *Emotion in the Human Face: Guidelines for Research and an Integration of Findings* (Elmsford, N.Y.: Pergamon, 1972), p. 107.

10. G. Simmel, "Sociology of the Senses: Visual Interaction," *Introduction to the Science of Sociology,* ed. R.E. Park and E.W. Burgess (Chicago: University of Chicago Press, 1921), p. 358.

11. Michael Argyle and Janet Dean, "Eye Contact Distance and Affiliation," *Sociometry* 28 (1965): 289-304.

12. G. Myers and M. Myers, *Dynamics of Human Communication,* p. 171.

13. D.C. Aguilera, "Relationships Between Physical Contact and Verbal Interaction Between Nurses and Patients," *Journal of Psychiatric Nursing* 5 (1967): 5-21.

14. Abne Eisenberg and Ralph Smith, *Nonverbal Communication,* pp. 66-67.

15. Albert Mehrabian, *Silent Messages* (Belmont, Calif.: Wadsworth Publishing Co., 1971), pp. 55-72.

16. Edward Hall, *Hidden Dimension* (Garden City, N.Y.: Doubleday & Co., 1966), pp. 1-6.

17. A.G. White, "The Patient Sits Down: A Clinical Note," *Psychosomatic Medicine* 15 (1953): 256-257.

18. Juluis Fast, *Body Language* (New York: Pocket Books, 1971), pp. 45-46.

19. Robert Sommer, "Studies in Personal Space," *Sociometry* 22 (1959): 247-260.

20. Edward Hall, *Silent Language* (New York: Fawcett Premier Book, 1959), pp. 163-164.

21. *Ibid.*

22. Ray Birdwhistell, "Background to Kinesics," *Etc: A Review of General Semantics* 13 (1955), 10-18.

SUGGESTED READINGS

Aguilera, D.C. "Relationships Between Physical Contact and Verbal Interaction Between Nurses and Patients." *Journal of Psychiatric Nursing* 5: 5-21.

Argyle, Michael, and Dean, J. "Eye Contact, Distance and Affiliation." *Sociometry* 23: 289-304.

Barnett, K.E. "The Development of a Theoretical Construct of the Concepts of Touch as They Relate to Nursing." Ph.D. Dissertation, North Texas State University, 1970.

Birdwhistell, Raymond. *Introduction to Kinesics.* Louisville: University of Louisville Press, 1970.

Casher, L., and Dixson, B.K. "The Therapeutic Use of Touch." *Journal of Psychiatric Nursing and Mental Health Services* 5: 442-451.

Ekman, P., and Friesen, W.V. "Head and Body Cues in the Judgment of Emotion: A Reformulation." *Perceptual and Motor Skills* 24: 711-724.

Felipe, N.J., and Sommer, R. "Invasions of Personal Space." *Social Problems* 14: 206-214.

Hall, Edward T. *The Silent Language.* Garden City, N.Y.: Doubleday & Co., 1959.

Knapp, Mark L. *Nonverbal Communication in Human Interaction.* New York: Holt, Rhinehart, and Winston, 1972.

Mahl, G.F. "Measuring the Patient's Anxiety During Interviews from Expressive Aspects of His Speech." *Transactions of the New York Academy of Sciences* 21: 249-257.

McCorkle, R. "Effects of Touch on Seriously Ill Patients." *Nursing Research* 23: 125-132.

Mehrabian, Albert. "Significance of Posture and Position in the Communication of Attitudes and Status Relationships." *Psychological Bulletin* 71: 359-372.

――――. "Nonverbal Betrayal of Feeling." *Journal of Experimental Research in Personality* 5: 64-73.

――――. "Communication Without Words." *Psychology Today* 2: 52-55.

Rosenfeld, H.M. "Approval Seeking and Approval Inducing Functions of Verbal and Nonverbal Responses in the Dyad." *Journal of Personality and Social Psychology* 4: 65-72.

Ruesch, J., and Kees, Weldon. *Nonverbal Communication.* Berkeley: University of California Press, 1956.

Sommer, Robert. *Personal Space: The Behavioral Basis of Design.* Englewood Cliffs, N.J.: Prentice Hall, 1969.

Watson, W.H. "The Meaning of Touch: Geriatric Nursing." *Journal of Communication* 25: 104-112.

White, A.G. "The Patient Sits Down: A Clinical Note." *Psychosomatic Medicine* 15: 256-257.

Zaidel, S.F., and Mehrabian, A. "The Ability to Communicate and Infer Positive and Negative Attitudes Facially and Vocally." *Journal of Experimental Research in Personality* 3: 233-241.

NONVERBAL REVIEW PUZZLE

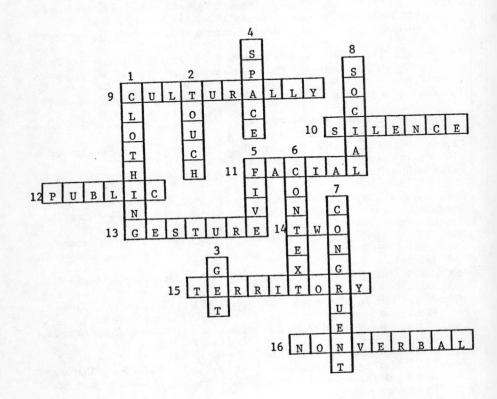

DOWN

1) An extension of self.
2) Most intimate of senses.
3) What you see is what you _____
4) One's territory.
5) Number of minutes it takes to form a first impression.
6) Nonverbal interpretation depends upon this.
7) Harmonious verbal and nonverbal messages.
8) A kind of distance, from 20 inches to five feet.

ACROSS

9) How nonverbal messages are learned.
10) A form of communication.
11) Expressions regarded as reliable indicators.
12) A kind of distance, from 5 to 100 feet.
13) A bodily action.
14) Number of basic types of messages sent at the same time.
15) We defend this.
16) The silent language.

Chapter 7

The Dynamics of the Nursing Staff's Effectiveness

CHAPTER OBJECTIVES

The purpose of this chapter is to enable you to CHANGE your communicative behavior in a *positive* direction. After studying the material you should be able to:

Communicate more effectively in small groups.

Have an understanding of group dynamics.

Assess and improve communication flow between nursing staff members, physicians, and patients.

Notice the differences between "supportive" and "defensive" group climates.

Gain new insights into the importance of group norms and roles.

Evaluate the quality of your work group in seven areas of group process.

At a recent national convention for nurses, a nurse stated: "We work best as a nursing team under conditions of severe stress. Suddenly something goes wrong and you can immediately sense everyone working together toward a common goal. Whether we like one another is immaterial. We have one goal and that goal is the welfare of the patient."

This statement should not surprise anyone. Most work groups tend to pull together toward a common goal when they are faced with conditions of severe stress. Group members realize the task cannot be accomplished unless everyone pulls together through total group cooperation.

Most of the time, however, nurses are not involved in such stressful situations. Thus, during their normal work periods, nursing teams are most vulnerable and do not achieve maximum productivity. The question then arises, How we can get members of the work team to work together under normal working conditions to the maximum of their ability?

Many important preplanned decisions on the nursing ward are made in earlier nursing staff meetings. Such preplanned decisions help determine what specific nursing decisions should be made during times of emergency. This type of prior group decision making is essential; small-group interaction enables nurses to discuss issues openly and frankly before emergencies arise. Such intragroup communication affects many members of the health care team—the surgeon, anesthesiologist, recovery room staff, nurses, staff members, and, ultimately, the patient—and provides opportunities for all staff members to discuss their feelings and gut level reactions to the issues at hand.

SMALL GROUP CHARACTERISTICS

A group is a collection of individuals who affect the character of the group and who are in turn affected by the group. The same people might react differently in one group than they do in another group. Delete one member from a group and the group's character changes; add another member and it will change again. In each case, the varied combinations of individual interests, abilities, and personalities produce a different group behavior.

The characteristics of a group are determined by the people comprising that group. Individuals join groups to satisfy their personal needs, but the needs of one person are not necessarily the same as those of another person, either in kind or degree. Moreover, people change from moment to moment; a person who is cooperative at one moment may be hostile at another.

Dorwin Cartwright and Alvin Zander define a group of people as an informal psychological group when the members interact chiefly through oral communication. More explicitly, an informal psychological group is

- a collection of two or more individuals
- who consciously identify with one another and
- interact dynamically,
- chiefly through the medium of oral communication,
- in such a way that all members are utilized to meet the satisfaction needs of each.[1]

This working definition should not lead one to believe that only oral communication is used in small group interaction. The term "interacting dynamically" infers the use of nonverbal communication as a vital part of the group process.

Nurses are involved predominantly in three types of interacting groups.

Learning Groups

Nurses in learning groups generally have some knowledge of the subject and are prepared for group meetings. The agenda of such groups is either consciously or unconsciously controlled. Nurses are personally involved in the discussion and strive to be objective. The main purpose of this type of group is to impart new information or knowledge to group members.

Policy-Making Groups

Policy-making groups are usually task-centered, have controlled agendas, are objective, and tend to proceed in a structured manner. Even though they are structured, they strive to retain a degree of spontaneity and informality. These groups establish nursing policy but are not responsible for the policy being carried out.

Decision-Making Groups

Decision-making groups are created to implement policies determined by policy-making groups. Their role is not to consider what should be policy but rather how to implement established policy. Such groups are highly task-oriented, usually operate under great pressure, and usually have rigidly controlled agendas.

THE DYNAMICS OF SMALL GROUPS

Sociologists and other theorists of small-group interaction have discovered that small groups take on character and personality, that they move through stages, just as individuals do, from infancy to maturity to death.

Group Status

Each member of a group contributes status and prestige to the group and develops additional status and prestige within the group. Because of their status or prestige, certain nurses assume responsibility for certain functions and are listened to more carefully by other group members.

Studies on member status within groups indicate that (1) high-status members tend to communicate more than low-status, (2) high-status members tend to communicate more with other high-status members, and (3) low-status members tend to communicate more with high-status members than with other low-status members.[2]

P.E. Slater discovered a high correlation between the rank of group members and the amount of talking they did within their group. High-status members gave the most information, received the most information, presented the best ideas, and gave guidance to the group's thinking.[3]

Group Norms

If rules are to be effective within a group, they must be accepted, and group members must know they are accepted by others as well as by themselves. These conditions create a group norm, defined as "shared acceptance of a rule."[4]

Group norms are normally instituted when the group is first formed. For example, if a nurse has called a group together, that nurse's attitudes, mannerisms, and so forth, will probably affect the development of the group's norms. If the group has a leader, the leader will also play an important role in establishing group norms. However, leaders cannot establish norms by themselves. Other high-status members of the group will also exert more influence upon group norms than average group members.

An interesting communication pattern develops in most groups. Psychology texts refer to this pattern as the "communicative pecking order" because the process is similar to the pecking order of chickens at feeding time, that is, one chicken eats first, followed by a second, and so on.

Thus, at the start of a meeting, the nurse who speaks first can greatly influence the standards of the group. The initial comments of that nurse may stimulate comments from others, and, before the group is aware of what has happened, group standards of participation have been established. On the other hand, the longer a nurse waits to contribute an idea or to share information, the more difficult it becomes for that nurse to speak and to influence the group.

When individuals with deviant attitudes attempt to violate group norms, social pressures are exerted upon the individuals to bring them into line. Social pressure is highest in groups that are highly cohesive. Thus, if a nurse expresses an opinion or uses language contrary to actions deemed acceptable, the group will concentrate its attention upon that nurse with a barrage of comment until the nurse gets back in line. If people persist in deviating from the group norm, the group will give up on them and often ignore them entirely until they come around or get out of the group.

Group norms can be changed, but this is a difficult task. Usually those who wish to change group norms must find support through changes in group personnel, in the excesses of established leaders, by external pressure for change, or through changes in the communication patterns of the group members. Sometimes, a group feels it is time for self-evaluation and decides through deliberative group effort to change some of the existing group norms.

Dean Barnlund and Franklin Haiman conclude,

> at least on the basis of present knowledge, that those members of a group who have more authority than the others (the leader, senior members, etc.), those who have disturbed personalities, and those who happen to get attention first are likely to be more influential in shaping group norms than the "average" member.[5]

Group Pressure

There is considerable evidence to indicate that individuals tend to conform to group standards, even when such standards contradict individual standards or beliefs. Solomon Asch conducted an experiment to examine the effect of group pressure on individual judgment. In each of his groups there were three trained subjects and one naive subject. All subjects were asked to judge which of two lines was longer. However, the trained subjects were instructed to say that the shorter line was longer. In most instances the trained subjects answered first, and then the naive subjects would go along with the majority view, regardless of their own perceptions.[6]

From this experiment it was generalized that in small groups the majority will tend to pull the minority to its point of view. Apparently people need to belong to such an extent that they will sacrifice their own opinions for those of the group.

Group Size

A group's ability to reach decisions, derive group satisfaction, and communicate efficiently is dependent upon the size of the group. George Beal, Joe Bohlen, and J. Neil Raudabaugh believe that the optimum size for small group efficiency is five members:

> (1) this size allows sufficient opportunity for each individual to participate and yet enough members are present to draw on for content and make it worthwhile; (2) there is not the possibility of a strict deadlock as with even numbers; (3) if the group splits it tends to split into a majority of 3 and a minority of 2, so that being in the minority does not isolate any one individual; (4) the group seems large enough for members to shift roles easily . . . and allows a member to easily withdraw from an awkward position.[7]

Most authorities tend to think that, as group size increases beyond five members, there is less group cohesiveness, a greater tendency toward more formal procedures, and increased difficulty in coordinating activities; and the group leader tends to talk to the group as a whole rather than to individual group members.

Slater reports that members of five-man groups expressed complete satisfaction with the size of their groups, indicating they were neither too large nor too small.[8]

As groups increase in size, subgroups form within the main group, and the number of interactions increases dramatically. This makes the task of structuring the group more difficult.

Robert Bostrom notes that in a dyad (two people) only two interactions are possible, A to B and B to A, but in a triad (three people) there are nine possibilities:[9]

A to B	B to C	A to B and C
A to C	C to B	B to A and C
B to A	C to A	C to A and B

He then shows the number of interactions that can take place in groups that range in size from two to eight members:[10]

Number in Group	Interactions Possible
2	2
3	9
4	28
5	75
6	186
7	441
8	1056

In summary, groups should be kept to a maximum size of five members, if at all possible. If there is a need to increase the size of the group, it would be best to form subgroups of five members to increase efficiency and member satisfaction. It should also be remembered that size, like leadership, is dependent upon the situation. A nursing work group, for example, may need to be larger than five. However, in general, five is the recommended size for a problem-solving group.

Group Setting

The setting in which nurses discuss problems and make group decisions is extremely important. The setting helps to establish the environmental climate in which the nursing group must work.

A seating arrangement in a circular or elliptical pattern in which everyone can be seen and no one is in a physically dominant position may help to create a more open and friendly atmosphere.[11] Such a seating arrangement allows each nurse to see and to respond to any other nurse in the group.

Barnlund concluded that eye contact is an important factor in spatial arrangements. In a study done in 1965, he found that, when interaction is desired, people seem to prefer to sit closer together and in a position in which eye contact is possible, rather than side by side, an arrangement that limits eye contact.[12]

Communication Networks

The four main communication networks employed by nursing groups are represented by the following figures:

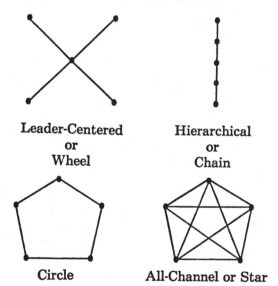

Leader-Centered
or
Wheel

Hierarchical
or
Chain

Circle

All-Channel or Star

Leader-Centered or Wheel

The wheel network allows the central person to communicate with any group member, and in turn the members must direct all their comments through the center. Harold Leavitt discovered that the central person in the wheel usually becomes the leader and enjoys that position much more than those on the periphery enjoy their positions.[13]

Hierarchical or Chain

The chain network allows people to talk to one or two group members but not to everyone in the chain. This reduces the opportunity for direct sharing of ideas and limits group satisfaction.

Circle

The circle network lends itself to high participation and usually results in high group-member satisfaction. At times, however, frustration can occur due to the fact that there is no central source of information.

All-Channel or Star

Most authorities agree that in the majority of cases, the all-channel or star pattern is the most suitable. Bill Conboy describes this design as the optimum arrangement for versatility and flexibility. It allows the maximum number of connections among members and provides freedom, involvement, and the greatest potential for reorganization. The group members can create almost any set of operating ground rules in order to achieve their goals. Neither the wheel nor the circle has this capacity for self-revision.[14]

Marvin Shaw summarized the findings of 18 group communication networks and concluded that "the wheel and the chain are better when the problem is simple. . . . However, when the problem is complex the decentralized networks such as the circle and all-channel are faster, more accurate, and result in higher member satisfaction."[15]

Group Goals

Many organizations have goals, but often the goals are unclear, nebulous, or unrealistic. Nurses must accept group goals in order for the group to achieve success, but the goals must also be closely related to the needs of individual group members.

Bobby Patton and Kim Giffin believe that the importance of goal specificity cannot be overemphasized. Their work has led them to conclude that groups fail, lose member commitment, bog down, and develop interpersonal dislikes because of a lack of specific goal identification.[16] Their point is that, if you aim for nothing in particular, it is likely you will achieve just that.

Behaviors That Cause Defensiveness

If one nurse has influence over another, within a group, it follows by definition that the nurse with the influence can bring about changes in the nurse being influenced. We see that the mere existence of a power relationship can and does, at times, pose a threat to the nurse being influenced, and we should expect that nurse to seek ways of defending against it.

Jack Gibb developed six categories that reflect behavior that arouses defensiveness and ultimately affects the climate of a work group.[17]

Evaluation: to question a person's values, standards, or motives. Even the simplest question may evoke defensiveness. This is a serious problem for nurses as they attempt to communicate with physicians and surgeons. The doctor's title reflects status, which can easily become a disruptive influence where cooperation is essential. The nurse has a need to question, to determine the needs of a patient, and only through a supportive climate of trust will the nurse feel free to question procedures or techniques. Questioning enables us to learn and grow and thus become more competent in our jobs.

Yet, at times remarks are made that have no malicious intent, but are interpreted that way. For example, how can a surgeon or physician ask, "Who did that?" and not be seen as accusing? We can overcome tendencies to evaluate or make such judgments within groups if we ask questions that are regarded as genuine requests for information. A nurse can be supportive by presenting feelings, events, perceptions, or processes that do not ask or imply that the receivers of the message change their behavior or attitudes.

Control: to try to do something to another, to attempt to change an attitude or behavior. If hidden motives are suspected, resistance is increased. The nurse can overcome this tendency by showing a desire to collaborate in defining a mutual problem and in seeking its solution.

Strategy: to make others think they are making their own decisions, and to make them feel that the speaker has a genuine interest in them. No one likes to be the victim of hidden motivation. Nurses in staff meetings should look for spontaneity rather than manipulation. Communicate with those who respond spontaneously, and in a straightforward and honest manner.

Neutrality: to express lack of concern for a fellow group member, to be clinical or detached from the feelings of the group. In the health care field we talk about TLC, "tender loving care," but do we exhibit this same degree of concern for our coworkers? How long has it been since you have told coworkers that you enjoy working with them and that they have made your job a little easier?

Nurses must learn to develop rapport with the people in their work group. They must be able to identify with the everyday problems of other group members, to share their feelings and accept their emotional values without making judgments about them. Neutrality can suggest indifference, and indifference breeds contempt. Whenever possible the nurse must combine understanding and empathy in dealing with another person's emotions, and make no attempt to change them. This type of emotional involvement makes the nurse supportive at the highest level.

Superiority: to communicate one's status as superior. For a group to be effective, its members must enjoy feelings of equality and work together on an equal basis to solve common group problems.

Certainty: to assume you have all the right answers. Nurses should develop attitudes of patience and try to avoid frozen judgments until all the evidence has been presented. Medical procedures are not employed until all of the diagnostic tests have been taken and analyzed. The same should be true of group decision making. Group members should be allowed to have their say and then, based on that information, an opinion may be formed.

Group Effectiveness

This chapter has attempted to show the various aspects of small group behavior that tend to make groups effective or ineffective. Therefore, the following comparisons can be made.[18]

Effective groups tend to have a high degree of permissiveness. This climate of permissiveness gives members an opportunity to speak their minds; they are inhibited only by normal restraints of tact, propriety and common sense. Members of ineffective groups exhibit the opposite behavior and act restrained during meetings. They leave the meeting muttering to themselves about the ideas they did not feel free to express. The effective group assigns tasks on the basis of people's skills and interests. The ineffective group assigns tasks with little thought or planning. Effective groups exhibit intergroup status where all members share in the recognition and rewards of group achievement. To become effective, groups need successes and from successes the group builds confidence and is able to meet new challenges.

To be an effective nursing group requires tremendous effort, but the satisfaction of group achievement will always be greater than that for individual achievement.

One last point should be made: In group meetings, too often we associate disagreement with personal dislike. Though people have difficulty disagreeing without being disagreeable, just because someone disagrees with us does not necessarily mean they dislike us.

Giffin and Patton state that disagreement on the nature of the problem or the value of a suggested solution is a necessary component of the process of group interaction, but that perceived personal dislike creates a negative, debilitating response. It is essential to discriminate accurately between disagreement and personal dislike if we are going to solve mutual problems cooperatively.[19]

The following test will help you to examine your own perceptions of the components of group effectiveness.

Group Effectiveness Questionnaire

This questionnaire examines your personal perception of the effectiveness of your nursing group, whether you are doing your job individually or working with other group members to meet a group goal. The questionnaire deals with seven parts of the group process: planning, problem solving/decision making, use of resources, responsibility, motivation/pride, communications, and climate.

Each part may be scored separately to determine the nursing group's strength or weakness in each of the process areas. The combined scores give a total group effectiveness score. Score each statement as follows: 1 = Strongly disagree. 2 = Disagree. 3 = Don't know or neutral. 4 = Agree. 5 = Strongly agree. The evaluative categories of the combined scores are shown at the end of the questionnaire.

Planning	Disagree			Agree	
(1) Our group goals are clearly defined.	1	2	3	4	5
(2) There is a high degree of commitment toward group goals.	1	2	3	4	5
(3) My group sets high standards of performance.	1	2	3	4	5
(4) The group does advance planning to avoid a crisis-like operating style.	1	2	3	4	5

(5) Our goals are well coordinated with other associated work groups and with higher organizational goals.   1 2 3 4 5

(6) Management asks for my ideas about better planning.   1 2 3 4 5

(7) When procedural changes are made or new equipment is placed in operation, my group is properly trained and prepared.   1 2 3 4 5

(8) Management provides adequate staffing.   1 2 3 4 5

Problem Solving/Decision Making	Disagree		Agree	

(9) My group develops several options before proposing a solution to a problem.   1 2 3 4 5

(10) In resolving group problems, each member of our group accepts a responsibility and constructively works toward resolution.   1 2 3 4 5

(11) We quickly resolve operational problems so that personal conflict does not build up.   1 2 3 4 5

(12) There is a general satisfaction concerning the quality of operational decisions that affect our group.   1 2 3 4 5

(13) Management accepts the consequences for a wrong decision and does not pass the blame to subordinates.   1 2 3 4 5

(14) If I have trouble on my job, I can count on my supervisor to be reasonable and to give the necessary assistance.   1 2 3 4 5

Use of Resources	Disagree		Agree	

(15) Group members utilize the skills of other members.   1 2 3 4 5

(16) There is adequate time and money to meet our important goals.   1 2 3 4 5

(17) The group displays a high level of technical or professional skill required for high performance.   1 2 3 4 5

(18) Our group meetings are action-oriented and productive.   1 2 3 4 5

(19) Members are efficient in how they spend their time.   1 2 3 4 5

(20) My job makes good use of my skills and abilities.   1 2 3 4 5

(21) People who get ahead in my department deserve to do so because of their high performance.   1 2 3 4 5

(22) When needed, we receive training in a timely manner.   1 2 3 4 5

Responsibility   Disagree   Agree

(23) Members of my group will go out of their way to help other members achieve their goals.   1 2 3 4 5

(24) Members of my group know each other's assignments and responsibilities.   1 2 3 4 5

(25) Members of our group follow through on assignments.   1 2 3 4 5

(26) My job gives me the chance to learn new skills and techniques.   1 2 3 4 5

(27) My job allows me to identify and solve problems on my own.   1 2 3 4 5

(28) Through discussion with management I can influence the decisions that affect my job.   1 2 3 4 5

(29) My group accepts the consequences when we make the wrong decision.   1 2 3 4 5

(30) My group actively looks for better ways to get the job done.   1 2 3 4 5

(31) I have a personal sense of responsibility to help my hospital be profitable.   1 2 3 4 5

Motivation/Pride   Disagree   Agree

(32) We have a record of success in our group that provides a sense of pride.   1 2 3 4 5

(33) There is general group satisfaction about   1 2 3 4 5
our contribution to the survival and
future success of our hospital.

(34) Employee benefits are very good.   1 2 3 4 5

(35) My department recognizes those who   1 2 3 4 5
consistently show high performance.

(36) I am making satisfactory progress   1 2 3 4 5
toward my career goals.

(37) What happens to my hospital is impor-   1 2 3 4 5
tant to me.

(38) I take personal pride in doing my job   1 2 3 4 5
well.

Communications	Disagree			Agree	

(39) My group enjoys an open, honest, and   1 2 3 4 5
direct style of communication.

(40) Disagreements are handled constructive-   1 2 3 4 5
ly, and we learn from the discussion.

(41) Members of my group effectively obtain,   1 2 3 4 5
through a variety of sources, sufficient
information to carry out their responsibilities.

(42) People at the top keep me advised of   1 2 3 4 5
proposed solutions to problems existing
at my level.

(43) My supervisor is aware of problems   1 2 3 4 5
existing at my level.

(44) Management gives credit and recogni-   1 2 3 4 5
tion to people who do a good job.

(45) I clearly understand the employee   1 2 3 4 5
benefits available to me.

Climate	Disagree			Agree	

(46) Members of my group have a high   1 2 3 4 5
degree of respect for the competence
and ability of the other members.

(47) My immediate supervisor treats everyone   1 2 3 4 5
fairly.

(48) I can honestly disagree with manage-   **1 2 3 4 5**
ment without fear of reprisal.

(49) Members of my work group trust each   **1 2 3 4 5**
other.

(50) I feel that management will fairly   **1 2 3 4 5**
represent my interests on issues con-
cerned with pay and working conditions.

TOTAL SCORING: 225–250 Superior, 175–224 Excellent, 125–174
Average, 75–124 Fair, 0–74 Poor.

Appendix 7-A

Suggested Activities

1. Ask each member of a nurses' group to draw an organizational chart for a hypothetical health care organization and to include in it the formal lines of authority and control. Next, ask the nurse to draw a hypothetical organizational chart that represents the informal lines of communication that might exist within the organization. Note the differences in the two charts. Does one permit a smoother communication flow? Does one increase employee morale? Does one make the organization more efficient? Obtain a copy of the actual organizational chart that your organization uses and analyze it to see if it can be improved.

2. Describe from a communication point of view the reasons for the many differences, disagreements, chaos, fights, and other divisions that occur in many organizational meetings today. Are we really having a breakdown of communication?

3. Bring to a meeting of five to seven nurses a jar of tongue depressors that have been broken in half. Count the number in the jar before you bring it in. Ask each nurse in the group to guess the number and to write it down on a piece of paper and put it away. Then ask the members of the group to come up with their best single estimate of the number of broken tongue depressors in the jar. The estimate must be derived by group consensus and not by group averaging or voting. In other words, the nurses should try to reason with and influence each other. After the group reaches a consensus, compare the group estimate with the individual guesses that were made earlier by each nurse. Which estimates were closest to the actual number of broken tongue depressors in the jar: the group's or the individual guesses? Are five to seven minds better than one mind? Do groups always make better decisions than isolated individuals? Is the sharing of information useful to a group?

SMALL GROUP REVIEW PUZZLE

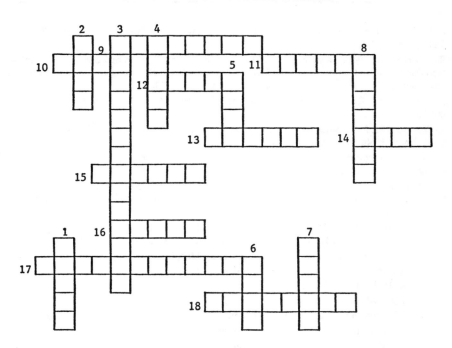

DOWN

1) A group must have these.
2) What status do members have who present the best ideas?
3) Effective groups have a high degree of this.
4) Number of people in a triad.
5) Affects the ability of groups to reach decisions.
6) The best type of network for most purposes.
7) A hierarchical network.
8) A group's environmental conditions.

ACROSS

9) Affected by group decisions.
10) Ideal group size.
11) One's position in a group.
12) Specific types of individual behavior exhibited by a group member.
13) Every group needs one of these.
14) Number of possible interactions in a group of eight people.
15) A network with no central source of information.
16) Shared acceptance of a rule.
17) Group togetherness.
18) One type of group.

(Answers are on page 124.)

NOTES

1. Dorwin Cartwright and Alvin Zander, *Group Dynamics* (New York: Harper & Row Publishers, 1968), pp. 46–48.

2. J.I. Hurwitz, A.F. Zander, and B. Hymovitch, "Some Effects of Power on the Relationships Among Group Members," *Group Dynamics*, ed. D. Cartwright and A. Zander (New York: Harper & Row Publishers, 1968), pp. 291–297.

3. P.E. Slater, "Role Differentiation in Small Groups," *American Sociological Review* 20 (1955): 303.

4. Theodore M. Newcomb, Ralph H. Turner, and Phillip E. Converse, *Social Psychology* (New York: Holt, Rhinehart, and Winston, Inc., 1965), p. 254.

5. Dean C. Barnlund and Franklin S. Haiman, *The Dynamics of Discussion* (Boston: Houghton Mifflin Co., 1960), pp. 199–200.

6. Solomon E. Asch, "Effects of Group Pressure Upon the Modification and Distortion of Judgments," *Readings in Social Psychology*, ed. G. Swanson, et al. (New York: Holt, Rhinehart, and Winston, 1952), pp. 2–11.

7. George M. Beal, Joe M. Bohlen, and J. Neil Raudabaugh, *Leadership and Dynamic Group Actions* (Ames, Iowa: Iowa State University Press, 1962), pp. 117–118.

8. P.E. Slater, "Contrasting Correlates of Group Size," *Sociometry* 21 (1958): 129–139.

9. Robert Bostrom, "Patterns of Communicative Interaction in Small Groups," *Speech Monographs* 37 (1970): 257.

10. *Ibid.*, p. 258.

11. Beal, Bohlen, and Raudabaugh, *Leadership and Dynamic Group Actions*, p. 81.

12. Dean C. Barnlund, *Interpersonal Communication: Survey and Studies* (Boston: Houghton Mifflin Co., 1968), pp. 559–560.

13. Harold Leavitt, "Some Effects of Certain Communication Patterns on Group Performance," *Journal of Abnormal and Social Psychology* 46 (1951): 38–50.

14. Bill Conboy, *Working Together: Communication in a Healthy Organization* (Columbus, Ohio: Charles E. Merrill Publishing Co., 1976), p. 31.

15. Marvin E. Shaw, "Communication Networks," *Advances in Experimental Social Psychology*, vol. 1, ed. Leonard Berkowitz (New York: Academic Press, 1964), pp. 111–147.

16. Bobby R. Patton and Kim Giffin, *Problem Solving Group Interaction* (New York: Harper & Row Publishers, 1973), pp. 147–148.

17. Jack R. Gibb, "Defensive Communication," *Journal of Communication* 11 (1961): 141–148.

18. R. Victor Harnack and Thorrel B. Fest, *Group Discussion Theory and Technique* (New York: Appleton-Century-Crofts, 1964), pp. 177–181.

19. Patton and Giffin, *Problem Solving Group Interaction*, p. 259.

SUGGESTED READINGS

Applbaum, Ronald L.; Bodaken, Edward M.; Sereno, Kenneth K.; and Anatol, Karl. *The Process of Group Communication.* Chicago: Science Research Associates Inc., 1979.

Aronoff, Joel, and Messe, Lawrence A. "Motivational Determinants of Small Group Structure." *Journal of Personality and Social Psychology* 17: 319-324.

Bales, Robert F. *Interaction Process Analysis.* Reading, Mass.: Addison-Wesley, 1950.

Bavelas, A. "Communication Patterns in Task Oriented Groups." *Journal of Acoustical Society of America* 22: 725-730.

Bradford, Leland P. *Group Development.* La Jolla, Calif.: University Associates, Inc., 1974.

Cartwright, Darwin, and Zander, Alvin, eds. *Group Dynamics.* New York: Harper & Row, Publishers, 1968.

Combs, A.W.; Avila, D.L.; and Purkey, W.W. *Helping Relationships Basic Concepts for the Helping Professions.* Boston: Allyn and Bacon, 1971.

Conboy, Bill. *Working Together: Communication in a Healthy Organization.* Columbus, Ohio: Charles E. Merrill Publishing Co., 1976.

Epstein, Charlotte. *Effective Interaction in Contemporary Nursing.* Englewood Cliffs, N.J.: Prentice Hall, Inc., 1974.

Hare, Paul A., and Larson, Carl E. "Seating Position and Small Group Interaction." *Sociometry* 26: 480-486.

Jacobs, Alfred, ed. *The Group as Agent of Change.* New York: Human Science Press, 1974.

Leth, Pamela C., and Vandemark, JoAnn F. *Small Group Communication.* Menlo Park, Calif.: Cummings Publishing Co., Inc., 1977.

Pfeiffer, J. William, and Jones, John E. *A Handbook of Structured Experiences for Human Relations Training,* vols. 1-6. Iowa City, Iowa: University Associates Press, 1973-1977.

Phillips, Gerald M., and Erickson, Eugene C. *Interpersonal Dynamics in the Small Group.* New York: Random House, 1970.

Roberts, K.H., and O'Reilly, C.A. "Failures in Upward Communication in Organizations: Three Possible Culprits." *Academy of Management Journal* 17: 205-215.

Rosenfeld, H., and Rosenfeld, A. *Human Interaction in the Small Group Setting.* Columbus, Ohio: Charles E. Merrill Publishing Co., 1973.

Sattler, William M., and Miller, N. Edd. *Discussion and Conference.* Englewood Cliffs, N.J.: Prentice Hall Inc., 1968.

Schien, E.H., and Bennis, W.G. *Personal and Organizational Change Through Group Methods.* New York: John Wiley and Sons Inc., 1965.

Tubbs, Stewart L. *A Systems Approach to Small Group Interaction.* Reading, Mass.: Addison-Wesley Publishing Co., 1978.

SMALL GROUP REVIEW PUZZLE

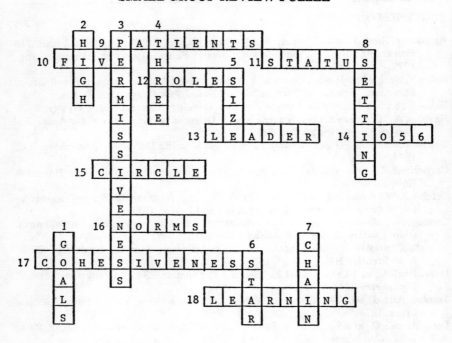

DOWN

1) A group must have these.
2) What status do members have who present the best ideas?
3) Effective groups have a high degree of this.
4) Number of people in a triad.
5) Affects the ability of groups to reach decisions.
6) The best type of network for most purposes.
7) A hierarchical network.
8) A group's environmental conditions.

ACROSS

9) Affected by group decisions.
10) Ideal group size.
11) One's position in a group.
12) Specific types of individual behavior exhibited by a group member.
13) Every group needs one of these.
14) Number of possible interactions in a group of eight people.
15) A network with no central source of information.
16) Shared acceptance of a rule.
17) Group togetherness.
18) One type of group.

Chapter 8

Barriers to Nursing Effectiveness

CHAPTER OBJECTIVES

The purpose of this chapter is to enable you to CHANGE your communicative behavior in a *positive* direction. After studying the material you should be able to:

Construct clearer messages.

Heighten your ability to diagnose and prescribe proper treatment for communicative illness.

Avoid communication breakdowns due to semantic differences.

Note the differences between signs and symbols.

Gain an awareness of the important differences between the verbal and situational context of messages.

Eliminate message distortion.

The health care industry today employs close to 5 million people and accounts for ten percent of our gross national product. The medical achievements are indeed impressive. Great progress has been made against a variety of diseases. Medical science has been able to virtually eliminate smallpox and polio. Rapid advances are being made to conquer cancer and heart disease. This type of medical progress demands clear and concise communication between health care practitioners. For such progress to continue, communication barriers must be recognized and eliminated. Yet, as the health care community continues to grow, there is a need for more communication, not less. More sources have to be tapped and more people informed. Information must move through many channels before reaching its intended destination. Thus, the communication flow lends itself to misinterpretation and sometimes poor communication.

BARRIERS

Addison Bennett attempted to substantiate the assumption that certain kinds of barriers exist in health care organizations. The hypothesis was tested in a survey of 326 hospital managers who returned the mailed questionnaire. Analysis showed that the type, size, or location (rural or urban) of the hospital did not significantly influence the nature of the comments.[1]

Bennett reported that seven barriers were listed by at least ten percent of the 326 hospital managers responding to the survey:[2]

Barrier Cited	Number of Mentions*	Percent Mentioning
(1) Poor Communication	145	44%
(2) Absence of Training	136	42
(3) Lack of Goals	93	29
(4) Lack of Coordination	76	23
(5) Time Constraints and Work Pressures	53	16
(6) Management Attitudes	52	16
(7) Medical Staff Attitudes	31	10

* The majority of respondents commented on more than one barrier.

PEOPLE MEANING

How many times have we heard someone say, "I don't remember exactly what I said, but I know what I meant." Poor communication is the result of misinterpretation and misunderstanding. When we believe that words have meaning, we are in serious trouble as communicators. If words mean something, try to interpret the following statement: "I was riding down the highway bareback and I was stopped by a big hat who thought I was a big rigger, but I was really a maniac who used to work on bumble bees."

If words mean something, this statement should contain meaning for you. But, for communication to be classified as "good," there must be a common code between the sender and receiver of the message. Thus, as shown in the cited statement, words do not mean, people mean; the meaning is in the person. In order to communicate effectively, we must have the same communicative code.

The statement you tried to interpret came from a truck driver Dictionary. Riding down the highway "bareback" means riding in the truck without the trailer behind it. To be stopped by a "big hat" means to be stopped by a state trooper. A "big rigger" is an arrogant truck driver. A "maniac" is a shop mechanic, and to work on "bumble bees" means to work on one-cycle engines.

Too many times assumptions are made that create communication barriers. We assume that words have meaning and that people have the same past experiences. However, the differing past experiences of people and the multiple meanings of most words make it easy to misinterpret or misunderstand the messages of others.

SIGNS AND SYMBOLS

A special area of study called semantics is concerned with the meaning of words, that is, with the relationship between a symbol and the thing it represents, called a referent.

We use both signs and symbols to communicate. An important distinction between the two is that signs "indicate" and symbols "represent." Patients who cough, tremble, or cry out in pain are exhibiting signs indicating that they are in distress. Nurses and physicians are constantly looking for signs in blood pressure, color of the skin, pupils of the eye, heart beat, and so on.

When nurses or physicians verbalize these signs, they use symbols. The use of symbols is one of the basic characteristics that separates humans from animals. Humans can use symbols but animals cannot; animals can only use signs.

Gail and Michelle Myers note that

> Symbols in a way are shortcuts. Imagine what it would be like if we did not have convenient shortcuts like words to communicate with one another. If I wanted to tell you something, anything at all, about an object and did not have words to name it, I would have to point to it so you would know what exactly I had in mind. Our conversation would be limited necessarily to the objects of persons or events actually present to our senses at the moment of conversation. If we did not have words at our disposal we would be extremely limited indeed. Actually we would not be much different from the animals whose survival depends upon getting around to get food, and whose communication is limited to groans and grunts.[3]

Fortunately, this condition does not hold for humans. We have developed words that enable us to communicate symbolically with one another. Imagine the dilemma of operating room nurses if there were no words to describe a particular surgical instrument and surgeons, grunting and groaning, had to look at and point to every instrument they needed.

Don Fabun estimates that there are 600,000 words in the English language today. The number is constantly growing, and new expressions are constantly being coined. The number of words an adult uses in daily conversation (aside from technical words associated with a profession) is about 2,000.[4]

Sanford Berman discovered that the 500 words used the most in the English language have at least 14 thousand different definitions.[5]

There are about 300 million English-speaking people in the world today and as they go about their daily lives, each of them has different experiences. Yet, even though their experiences differ, they have the same basic store of accepted symbols to use in reporting to each other what they have experienced. Each symbol must, therefore, be used to cover a wide range of meanings.[6]

Nursing schools have certain basic common programs with respect to content. However, the individual ability of each teacher and student is a key determinant of what the students learn and of their ability to apply what they learn within a hospital setting. No two nurses are alike, no two nurses have the same training, and no two nurses have the same personality or motivation. Each is unique, and it is this uniqueness that determines the personal interpretation of communicative messages.

THE FALLACY OF WORD MEANING

Many times we miscommunicate because we mistakenly think the word we are using has one universal meaning, that it will mean the same to someone else as it does to us. A story from Lewis Carroll's *Alice's Adventures in Wonderland* points up the fallacy that words have meaning:

> "I don't know what you mean by 'glory,'" Alice said. Humpty Dumpty smiled contemptuously. "Of course you don't till I tell you. I mean there is a nice knockdown argument for you." "But glory does not mean a nice knockdown argument," Alice objected. "When I use a word," Humpty Dumpty said in a rather scornful tone, "it means just what I choose it to mean—neither more nor less." "The question is," said Alice, "whether you can make words mean so many different things." "The question is," said Humpty Dumpty, "who is to be master, that's all."[7]

In this case Humpty Dumpty was assuming, in his arrogant way, that the meaning the word held for him would have the same meaning for Alice. He was also strongly suggesting that the word had "better" mean the same to Alice or else she would have to answer to him. This is the type of attitude and belief that hinders the sharing of ideas and the transfer of information.

Perhaps the mistaken belief that words have meaning stems from what Irving Lee calls the "container myth:"

> If you think of words as vessels, then you are likely to talk about the meaning of a word as if the meaning were "in" that word. Assuming this, it is easy to endow words with characteristics. Just as you might say that one vessel is costlier or more symmetrical than another, you may say that one word is intrinsically more suitable for one purpose than another, or that, in and of itself, a word will have this or that meaning rather than any other. When one takes this view, he seems to say that meaning is to a word as contents are to a container.[8]

Obviously words do not contain meaning. Rather the meaning is in the person; words in differing contexts hold different meanings for the users of those words. For instance:

- Dog: A canine animal.
- Dog: To loaf on the job.
- Dog: A clamp used on a lathe.
- Dog: To follow closely.
- Dog: A kind of sandwich.
- Dog: An andiron used in a fireplace.

MESSAGE CONTEXT

A nurse must be able to discriminate accurately between the "verbal" and "situational" contexts of messages. Nurse A tells Nurse B about a patient. Nurse B receives the verbal context of the message and thus sees the patient's medical condition through the past experiences of Nurse A. Later, when Nurse B decides to check on the patient through direct observation, the situation might be entirely different from the one that was verbalized by Nurse A. Now Nurse B can see and talk to the patient, check medication cards, and so on, and thereby have a better understanding of the situation and how to respond to it.

This is not to say that messages should not be verbalized or passed from one source to another. But, when a situation is one of utmost importance, it should be recognized that conditions of the situation are not always the way they have been verbalized.

The following two stories underscore the point that to communicate effectively we must use language that has a common meaning for both sender and receiver and that is sent and received in its proper context.

The Stomach Operation

"Have you ever had an operation on your stomach before?" the doctor at Mt. Pleasant Hospital asked the patient. "No sir," the patient replied. Still, just to be sure, the doctor decided to take a few x-rays of the patient's stomach. The x-rays disclosed that the patient had only about half of his stomach left. "I thought you said that you had never had an operation on your stomach before," the doctor said firmly. "I didn't," the patient replied, "I was on my back."

Cleaning Pipes

A plumber wrote to a government agency, "I find that hydrochloric acid quickly opens pipes. Is this a good thing to use?" A scientist at the agency replied, "The efficacy of hydrochloric acid is indubitable, but the corrosive residue is incompatible with metallic permanence."

The plumber wrote back, thanking him for the assurance that hydrochloric acid was all right. Disturbed by this turn of events, the scientist showed the letter to his boss, another scientist, who then wrote to the plumber himself, "We cannot assume responsibility for the production of toxic and noxious residue with hydrochloric acid and suggest you use an alternative procedure."

The plumber wrote back that he agreed, the hydrochloric acid worked fine. Now greatly disturbed by these misunderstandings, the scientists took the problem to their top boss. He broke the jargon and wrote to the plumber, "Don't use hydrochloric acid; it eats the hell out of pipes!"

TECHNICAL USE OF WORDS

The technical use of words, as the preceding examples indicate, can result in miscommunication. Operating room nurses are extremely sensitive to this fact. Not all surgeons use the same terms for what are essentially the same surgical instruments. One of the first things operating room nurses do when they change hospitals is to find out what terms the surgeons use for their surgical instruments. People can communicate clearly only if they are using the same communicative code.

Have you ever wondered why a doctor says "neoplasm" instead of "cancer" or "myocardial infarction" instead of "heart attack?" According to Saul Radovsky, a suburban Boston doctor, the lingo helps to preserve the mystery of medicine. He notes that "sometimes doctors use words so obscure that even other medical people cannot understand them."[9]

Radovsky, in outlining his theory of why doctors write so poorly, gave the example of two researchers who wrote about a test they performed while attempting to learn why a boy's blood was infected:

> We used a chemiluminescence assay to examine the patient's polymorphonuclear leukocyte responses to numerous particulate and soluble stimuli. The patient's polymor-

phonuclear leukocytes had substantially depressed chemiluminescent responses during phagocytosis of opsonized particles.[10]

The researchers were explaining that the patient's white blood cells were not generating the usual amount of light when they attacked foreign invaders in the bloodstream.

There is obviously a need for technical language, but at times it can be overused. Technical language enables two people to communicate quickly and concisely, but only to the extent that both have the same code. When they have the same code, they have a common understanding, and their messages are being transferred and interpreted as they were intended to be transferred and interpreted.

Nurses should not be asked if they understand. This is especially true with respect to communications between a supervisor and an employee. When supervisors ask subordinates if they understand, the pressure is on the subordinates to respond affirmatively; the question calls for a predisposed answer. If they respond negatively, the subordinates may feel that their supervisors will think they are ignorant. If they respond positively, their supervisors will think they understand when in fact they may not.

Rather than "Do you understand?" ask, "What do you understand?" This forces the receiver of the message to repeat the message to the satisfaction of the sender, thereby ensuring a common understanding.

As mentioned earlier, words hold different meanings for different people. The multiple meanings that people attach to words can at times create embarrassing situations, as, for example, in the following supposedly true story:

A man walked into a doctor's office and the receptionist asked him what he had. He said, "Shingles." So she took his medical history, height, and weight and told him to wait. A half-hour later a nurse came in and asked him what he had. He said, "Shingles." So she took his blood pressure, gave him a blood test, an electrocardiogram, and told him to take off his clothes and wait for the doctor. A half-hour later the doctor came in and asked what he had. He said, "Shingles." The doctor asked, "Where?" He said, "Outside in the truck; where do you want them."

An anonymous poet wrote the following:

Remember when hippie meant big in the hips,
And a trip involved travel in cars, planes, and ships?

When pot was a vessel for cooking things in,
And hooked was what grandmother's rugs may have
been?
When fix was a verb that meant mend or repair,
And be-in meant merely existing somewhere?
When neat meant well organized, tidy and clean,
And grass was ground cover, normally green?
When groovy meant furrowed with channels and hollows?
And birds were winged creatures, like robins and
swallows?
When fuzz was a substance, real fluffy, like lint,
And bread came from bakeries and not from the mint?
When roll meant a bun, and rock was a stone,
And hang-up was something you did with the phone?
It's groovy man, groovy, but English it's not.
Methinks our language is going to pot.

We can avoid miscommunicating if we remember these points:

- Words have no meaning.
- Meaning is in the person.
- People should not be word-minded.
- They should be person-minded.
- Messages should be questioned and paraphrased.
- People should seek feedback.

MESSAGE DISTORTION

When messages are passed from one person to another, there is a tendency for the message to become distorted. One of the weaknesses of the chain communication network discussed in Chapter 5 is that, as messages are passed from one person to the next, distortion takes place, some information is lost, and new information is added. Each person in the chain interprets the message somewhat differently and passes on the new interpretation. When the message reaches the end of the chain it often barely resembles the original message. Consider the following:

- **The colonel to the executive officer:** "Tomorrow evening at approximately 2000 hours, Halley's Comet will be visible in this area, an event that occurs only once every 75 years. Have the men fall out in the battalion area in fatigues and I will explain the rare phenomenon to them. In case of rain, we will not be able to see anything, so march the men into the theatre and I will show them films of it."

- **The executive officer to the company commander:** "By order of the Colonel, tomorrow at 2000 hours, Halley's Comet will appear above the battalion area. If it rains, fall the men out in fatigues, then march to the theatre where the rare phenomenon will take place, something which occurs every 75 years."
- **The company commander to the lieutenant:** "By order of the Colonel in fatigues at 2000 hours tomorrow evening, the phenomenal Halley's Comet will appear in the theatre. In case of rain in the battalion area, the Colonel will give another order, something which occurs once every 75 years."
- **The lieutenant to the sergeant:** "Tomorrow at 2000 hours, the Colonel will appear in the theatre with Halley's Comet, something which happens every 75 years if it rains. The Colonel will then order the Comet into the battalion area."
- **The sergeant to the squad:** "When it rains tomorrow at 2000 hours, the phenomenal 75-year-old General Halley, accompanied by the Colonel, will drive his Comet through the battalion area theatre in fatigues."

On a more serious note, the preceding illustration has some parallels to a situation in which a doctor prescribes medicine for a patient. Very often, patients do not understand their doctors' drug prescriptions and procedures. Much of this misunderstanding could be avoided if physicians prescribed fewer drugs, gave less complex medication schedules, and made a greater effort to ensure that their patients understood the procedure to be followed when taking the medication. As the directions become more complex, the chances of distortion and error are increased.

AN IMPORTANT DISTINCTION

As we move toward the end of the twentieth century, communication gets blamed increasingly whenever something goes wrong. A popular refrain is, "We had a communication breakdown." At times this is obviously true, but at other times apparently "good" communication indeed turns out to be "poor" communication.

The key to this perceptual dilemma lies in the word "meaning." The goal of every communicative act is the transfer of a common meaning between the sender and the receiver of the message. However, at times we may be reprimanded or offered constructive criticism that we do not fully appreciate. It is at such moments that we are likely to say, "We had a communication breakdown" when, in fact, there was no breakdown at all. The common meaning was there, the communicative act was clear, but our displeasure evoked a response of poor communication when the communication could not have been clearer.

It is thus important to be able to distinguish between good communication with a common understanding and poor communication with little or no understanding.

Appendix 8-A

Suggested Activities

PURPOSE OF THE EXERCISE

This activity is designed to demonstrate individual differences in perception. The different meanings attached to the questions and the responses to the list of words reinforce the basic theme, "meanings are in people." Our perceptions are based on "our" experiences, "our" present motivation, and they determine how "we" interpret the messages of others.

DIFFERING REFERENTS

Read each statement and its accompanying question to a group of nurses and ask them to write down their answers. When you have completed the questions, ask some of the nurses to read their answers to the group.

1. The doctor was middle aged. How old was he?
2. A nurse had an average income. What was the nurse's income?
3. The nurses had a few drinks. How many did they each have?
4. She was carrying an armload of bandages. How many bandages did she carry?
5. It was a typical hospital. What was it like?
6. The nurse was average height. How tall is that?

THE USE OF SYMBOLS

Ask a group of nurses to draw four columns on a piece of 8½-by-11-inch paper. Ask each to write the label "symbols" at the top of the column on the left-hand side of the page. The remaining three columns should be labeled, "favorable," "unfavorable," and "neutral." The paper should look like this:

Symbols	Favorable	Unfavorable	Neutral

Explain to the group that you will read a word which should be written in the column labeled "symbols." The nurses should then put a check in the column (favorable, unfavorable, or neutral) which best describes their individual reaction to the word. After all the words have been read, poll the nurses on several of the words to determine individual differences in perception.

Here is a suggested list of words. You may, of course, use any other list of words which suits your purpose:

Symbol	Favorable	Unfavorable	Neutral
(1) Student Nurse			
(2) Registered Nurse			
(3) Physician			
(4) Night Duty			
(5) Payroll Office			
(6) Overtime			
(7) Intern			
(8) Patient			
(9) Hospital Cafeteria			
(10) Performance Appraisal			

MESSAGE TRANSMISSION

This exercise can be used to illustrate how messages become distorted as information is passed from one person to another. Divide the total group into subgroups of five to seven nurses each. Choose three members from each subgroup, designated Nurse A, Nurse B, and Nurse C. The three members from each subgroup should then leave the room.

Show a picture to the remaining members of the subgroups. Give each subgroup five minutes to redraw the picture and write a description of it.

Each subgroup will then call in its own Nurse A, and describe the picture. Nurse A may not ask questions but may ask the subgroup to repeat the description once. Nurse A may not write down the description or attempt to draw the picture as it is described.

The subgroup will then call in Nurse B. In front of the subgroup, Nurse A must tell Nurse B what the subgroup described. Nurse B may not ask questions but may ask Nurse A to repeat the description once. Nurse B may not write down the description or attempt to draw the picture as it is described. Nurse A may now rejoin the subgroup.

The subgroup will then call in Nurse C. In front of the subgroup, Nurse B must tell Nurse C what Nurse A said the subgroup described. Nurse C may not ask questions but may ask Nurse B to repeat the description once. Nurse C may not write down the description or attempt to draw the picture as it is described. Nurse B may now rejoin the subgroup.

Then ask Nurse C to go to the blackboard and draw and verbally explain the picture described by Nurse B. When Nurse C is finished, compare the drawing with the original picture drawn and described by the subgroup.

BARRIERS REVIEW PUZZLE

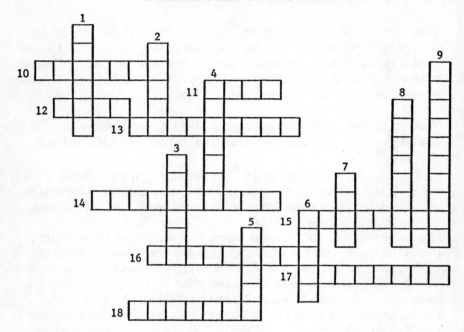

DOWN

1) Good communication always produces this type of meaning between people.
2) The employment of language.
3) Who has meaning?
4) What you should be sensitive to.
5) Indicates rather than represents.
6) Words have what type of usage?
7) Never ask, "Do you understand?" It is better to ask, "_____ do you understand?"
8) What represents a word symbol?
9) To check communication.

ACROSS

10) Words or things that stand for something not present.
11) Without this people have no meaning.
12) We miscommunicate because we think words have _____ usage.
13) The study of the meaning of words.
14) A communication barrier.
15) What communication conveys.
16) A type of word usage.
17) When communicating we should always seek to _____ meaning.
18) Do not think of words in this manner.

(Answers are on page 143.)

NOTES

1. Addison Bennett, "Toward More Effective Management: A Special Study in Management Problems and Practices," *Hospital Topics*, July, 1973, p. 15.
2. *Ibid.*
3. Gail Myers and Michelle Myers, *The Dynamics of Human Communication* (New York: McGraw Hill Book Co., 1973), p. 54.
4. Don Fabun, *Communications* (Beverly Hills, Calif.: The Glencoe Press, 1968), pp. 27–28.
5. Sanford Berman, *Understanding and Being Understood* (San Diego, Calif.: The International Communication Institute, 1965), p. 14.
6. Fabun, *Communications*, p. 28.
7. Lewis Carroll, *Alice's Adventures in Wonderland, Through The Looking Glass, and the Hunting of the Snark* (New York: Modern Library Inc., 1925), pp. 246–247.
8. Irving Lee, "On a Mechanism of Misunderstanding," *Promoting Growth Toward Maturity in Interpreting What Is Read*, ed. Gray (Chicago: University of Chicago Press, 1951), pp. 86–90.
9. Saul Radovsky, "Medical Writing: Another Look," *The New England Journal of Medicine* 301, no. 3, p. 134.
10. Saul Radovsky, *The New and Observer*, July 22, 1979, p. 21.

SUGGESTED READINGS

Berman, Sanford I. *Understanding and Being Understood.* San Diego: International Communication Institute, 1965.
Chase, Stuart. *The Power of Words.* New York: Harcourt, Brace, and World, Inc., 1954.
Fleishman, Alfred. *Sense and Nonsense: A Study in Human Communication.* San Francisco: International Society for General Semantics, 1971.
Frogman, Robert. "How to Say What You Mean; Business Communication." *Nation's Business* 45: 76–78.
———. "Prevent Short Circuits When You Talk." *Nation's Business* 51: 88–89.
———. "Make Words Fit the Job." *Nation's Business* 47: 76–79.
Hayakawa, S.I. *The Use and Misuse of Language.* New York: Fawcett World Library: Crest, Gold Medal, and Premier Books, 1962.
Heyel, C. "How to Communicate Better with Employees." *American Business Communication Bulletin* 37, no. 2: 38–40.
Johnson, Wendell. "The Fateful Process of Mr. A Talking to Mr. B." *Harvard Business Review* 31: 49–56.
Lee, Irving J. *How to Talk with People.* New York: Harper & Row, 1952.
———, and Lee, Laura L. *Handling Barriers in Communication.* New York: Harper & Row, 1957.
Minteer, Catherine. *Understanding in a World of Words.* San Francisco: International Society for General Semantics, 1970.
Ogden, C.K., and Richard, I.A. *The Meaning of Meaning.* New York: Harcourt, Brace and World, Inc., 1952.

Roethlisberger, Fritz J. "Barriers to Communication Between Men." *Northwestern University Information* 20, no. 25, April 21, 1952.

Rogers, Carl. "Communication: Its Blocking and Facilitation." *Northwestern University Information* 20, no. 25: 9–15.

Weaver, C.H. "Measuring Point of View as a Barrier to Communication." *Journal of Communication* 7, no. 1: 5–13.

Wiksell, Wesley. *Do They Understand You?* New York: McMillan and Co., 1960.

BARRIERS REVIEW PUZZLE

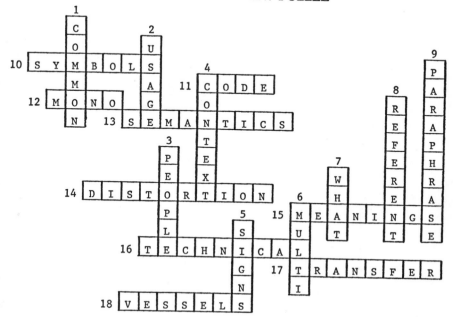

DOWN

1) Good communication always produces this type of meaning between people.
2) The employment of language.
3) Who has meaning?
4) What you should be sensitive to.
5) Indicates rather than represents.
6) Words have what type of usage?
7) Never ask, "Do you understand?" It is better to ask, "_____ do you understand?"
8) What represents a word symbol?
9) To check communication.

ACROSS

10) Words or things that stand for something not present.
11) Without this people have no meaning.
12) We miscommunicate because we think words have _____ usage.
13) The study of the meaning of words.
14) A communication barrier.
15) What communication conveys.
16) A type of word usage.
17) When communicating we should always seek to _____ meaning.
18) Do not think of words in this manner.

Chapter 9

The Nurse's Employment Interview

CHAPTER OBJECTIVES

The purpose of this chapter is to enable you to CHANGE your communicative behavior in a *positive* direction. After studying the material you should be able to:

Create a favorable impression during the employment interview.

Have a thorough understanding of the five stages of the employment interviewing process.

Anticipate the types of questions that may be asked.

Notice and respond to various interviewing techniques.

Gain access to employment services or job leads.

Eliminate common interviewing mistakes.

Registered nurses (R.N.s) exhibit a great deal of mobility during their lifetimes.[1] Many of their employment moves occur within the first few years of graduation from nursing school. As noted in Table 9-1, though most nurses take jobs in the same geographic area in which they graduated, they are likely to move to another area within a few years.

Nurses are almost as willing to make interstate as intrastate moves. As indicated in Table 9-2, the R.N.s most willing to move are the recently hired, single, separated, widowed, or divorced nurses, and those with no children and relatively little income from sources other than R.N. employment. When considering a move, nonfinancial incentives appear to appeal more to the single R.N. than financial incentives. On the other hand, separated, divorced, or widowed nurses are more likely to emphasize salary.[2]

This type of mobility makes it appropriate that we examine a specific form of interpersonal communication that is frequently used in organizational settings: the employment interview. Robert Goyer, Charles Redding and John Rickey describe interviewing as a form of

Table 9-1 R.N.s' Mobility: Interstate Moves

Stage of movement	Remained in same state	Remained in same census division but changed states	Changed census divisions	Total
Nursing school graduation to first job				
Yr. R.N. grad.				
1930-1939	87.2%	6.7%	6.1%	100.0%
1950-1959	85.0	6.5	8.5	100.0
1965-1969	83.2	5.4	11.4	100.0
First job to current job				
Yr. R.N. grad.				
1930-1939	55.7	11.5	32.8	100.0
1950-1959	57.0	13.6	29.3	100.0
1965-1969	61.1	11.6	27.3	100.0

Source: Department of Health, Education, and Welfare, 1975.

Table 9-2 The R.N.s' Willingness To Move to Another State

R.N. Group	Yes, for money	Yes, but not for money	No
Duration of current employment:			
Employed under 1 year	14.2%	16.5%	69.3%
Employed 1-5 years	13.9	13.9	72.2
Employed more than 5 years	6.5	6.1	87.3
Sex:			
Women	12.0	13.0	75.1
Men	30.6	23.6	45.8
Marital status:			
Single	21.6	27.2	51.3
Married, spouse present	7.7	9.0	83.3
Other (sep., wid., div.)	21.7	10.1	68.3
Children:			
Children, ages 0-6 only	10.4	10.6	79.0
Children, ages 7-18 only	9.8	5.3	84.9
Children, ages 0-18	8.8	5.4	85.8
None	15.8	19.0	65.2
Spouse earnings and income from other sources:			
$0-5,000	12.7	15.5	71.8
$5,001-10,000	8.9	9.3	81.8
$10,001-15,000	2.6	5.3	92.1
$15,001-25,000	5.1	7.8	87.1
$25,000 plus	5.5	5.5	89.0

Source: Department of Health, Education and Welfare, 1975.

dyadic interpersonal communication that involves two persons, at least one of whom has a preconceived and serious purpose, and both of whom speak and listen from time to time.[3] With this definition in mind, the following steps in the employment interviewing process can be examined.

HOW TO FIND THE RIGHT JOB

To avoid frustration and save you and your prospective employer time, you should develop a preliminary self-assessment of your qualifications and interests before applying for any job. A checklist of your interests and qualifications is an essential first step.

Identify Your Skills and Special Interests

- In what areas of nursing do you have experience? Do you prefer specific departments or duties where your skills and experience can best be utilized?
- Are you looking for career-expansion possibilities in a particular field of nursing?
- Which hospitals have openings in your specialty (emergency room, operating room, recovery room, medical, surgical and cardiac intensive care units, labor and delivery, obstetrics-gynecology, pediatrics, psychiatry, or physical therapy)?

Identify Your Personal Needs

- In which geographical areas do you wish to work? Are you restricted to any particular geographic area due to personal commitments? Will the job require additional time and expense in commuting?
- Do you need alternate shift schedules to meet family responsibilities or to enable you to pursue additional education?
- Does the prospective job provide opportunities for professional growth (inservice training programs, educational institutions in the area)? Is tuition provided for additional course work, and are staffing schedules adjusted to accommodate class hours?

Determine What Procedure to Follow

- For out-of-state jobs, contact the state board of nursing for information on the endorsement of your present license and other specific requirements. Another source of information may be the area nursing associations.
- Compare your initial checklist against available hospital openings. Make your selections and then arrange them in priority order.
- If possible, obtain information about a prospective place of employment by talking to nurses who work or have worked there. Remember that the grass always looks greener on the other side of the street. Another nurse may reject a hospital because of a particular philosophy or policy that is fully acceptable to you.

MAKING CONTACT

Since you will be applying to several hospitals for different reasons, your application letter should be "personalized." This means that the original covering letter should be neatly and freshly typed each time on 8½-by-11-inch, white bond paper with a 25 percent cotton fiber. A resume should accompany the application letter. The resume itself may be duplicated, preferably by Xerox or offset.

The Application Letter

The application letter should be in proper business form. Use the full name and title of the person being addressed. The letter should include the reasons for your application and also indicate that a resume has been enclosed. It should also suggest available times for an interview.

The Resume

The resume contains vital data about your education, experience, and skills. The resume, like the application letter, should be typed, but then it may be reproduced; it does not have to be freshly typed each time. It should be originally typed on 8½-by-11-inch, white bond paper with a 25 percent cotton fiber.

Set good-sized margins and triple space between each section. Place headings in capital letters along the left hand margin. List educational and work experiences chronologically in reverse order, the most recent education first and the most current position first. After titling the page and centering your name, address, and telephone number, organize your data in the following seven sections:

1. *License information:* Indicate the number, date, and state in which you are registered.
2. *Employment experience:* For each position, give the year, title, and position held, employer and address, description of duties, skills utilized, and responsibilities involved.
3. *Educational background:* Give the certificate or degree attained, the name and location of each school and the year you graduated or expect to graduate. If you have advanced credits, list them along with subjects you are currently taking. In a separate subsection, list extracurricular activities, inservice training, workshops, or conventions you have taken or attended.

4. *Additional skills and experience:* Attempt to personalize yourself in this section. Provide information on any volunteer work (in or out of nursing), civic contributions, and educational studies outside of nursing.

5. *Awards and prizes:* Cite any special recognition you have received at work or school.

6. *Professional membership:* List the professional groups you belong to, offices held, committee assignments, and so forth.

7. *Professional and personal references:* Carefully select three references whose permission to be used as references has been received, and list their full names, titles, and business addresses.

PREPARING FOR THE INTERVIEW

Most interviewers not only expect but welcome questions from you during the interview. Many of your questions will be concerned with hospital policy, procedures, and opportunities. It is usually best to group your questions into categories and then, during the interview, to deal with one category at a time. If you receive vague answers, do not hesitate to ask for clarification, without, however, appearing to be abrasive. Here are some typical questions grouped by category:

The Job

- Is the hospital accredited?
- What is the policy on performance appraisals? On promotions?
- What service specialties does the hospital offer?
- What does the orientation for new staff members cover and how long does it last?
- What is the procedure for transferring to other units?
- Are there job descriptions that clarify the duties and responsibilities of each staff job?

Administration of the Nursing Service

- Does each nursing unit conduct nursing care conferences?
- Does each nursing unit update its plans? Does it have written descriptions of care procedures? Does it have guidelines on the responsibilities of each shift?
- Are there written procedures for grievances? For emergencies? For evacuation?

Pay Scales and Shifts

- What is the starting salary?
- Are increments automatic (how often?) or according to merit? If by merit, what is the standard that is used?
- Are there pay differentials for weekend service, holidays, and overtime?
- How is the rotation shift arranged?
- Is sufficient notice given on time schedules?
- Is there any flexibility to accommodate personal needs or professional needs such as workshops, conventions, short courses, and so forth?

Educational Opportunities

- Is there an active inservice or continuing education program?
- Is the program held during each shift?
- Does the hospital provide tuition assistance for nurses registered in job-related studies at a college or university?
- Will the hospital consider such studies in determining raises or promotions?

Fringe Benefits

Most hospitals provide a booklet that spells out in detail the fringe benefits that are available to their employees. For example, most booklets contain information on vacation time, sick leave, employee health services, promotions, transfers, retirement, leaves of absence, and other policies affecting employees. Try to get a copy of this booklet before the interview and read it. Indeed, many of the questions in the categories cited above may be answered in material that you can obtain before the interview. In the interview, ask only those questions that are important to you and whose answers are not provided in the material you received previously from a prospective employer.

THE INTERVIEW

During the interview, it is important:

- to be punctual and dress conservatively
- to have a copy of your resume
- to have your social security number available

- to maintain eye contact with the interviewer
- to be direct in your answers, nonrepetitive in your questions, and honest in the discussion of your goals
- if offered the position, to request a tour of the facilities and especially the specific department you will be assigned to

William Brooks points out that the interviewer and the applicant cannot depend upon words alone. They must also be sensitive to nonverbal communication, to feelings and attitudes, to the interpersonal relationships that exist or are developing, and to their own accuracy and efficiency in *intrapersonal* communication.[4]

The interview may be regarded as having five parts or stages:

The Warmup Stage

It is essential to establish rapport quickly with the interviewer. E.C. Webster found that interviewers tend to form initial impressions about applicants within the first four or five minutes of the interview and that in the remaining time they search for additional information to support and substantiate their hunches.[5]

The Applicant-Talking Stage

As an applicant, you can expect to talk at least one-half the time during the interview. It is also important, however, that you receive information about the job. Only through this type of mutual information exchange can you make a sound decision. In this context, it is not uncommon for an interviewer's biases to determine the outcome of the interview. E.C. Mayfield notes that interviewers often disagree with one another quite radically; the candidate rated best by Interviewer A might be rated poorest by Interviewer B. Indeed, your future career might depend on which interviewer you happen to meet on the day of your interview.[6]

The Questioning Stage

The types of questions that may be asked will vary from interview to interview. However, Arthur Pell found that the following six kinds of questions are most frequently asked:[7]

1. *The "W" questions:* "What?" "When?" "Who?" "Why?" and "Where?"—coupled with "How?"—are types of questions used in

most interviewing situations. These are commonly referred to in the journalistic world as the 5 W's and H.

2. *Leading questions:* Leading questions may be used to control the interview. Such questions also often move applicants to give answers that they think the interviewer wants to hear. This trap should be avoided; applicants should be honest in their responses.

3. *Probing questions:* Incisive and specific probing questions are used to obtain additional details about a particular area. Probing questions are asked to see if applicants are familiar with the area being examined.

4. *"Yes" or "No" questions:* The closed yes-or-no type of question requires the applicant to respond in only one of two ways; it denies applicants the chance to expand their answers.

5. *Situational questions:* The interviewer can use situational questions to pose hypothetical problems and to encourage the applicant to answer. This type of question can be very helpful to the applicant because sometimes the question may not be wholly hypothetical. It may well concern problems presently existing in the hospital that the interviewer would like to know how the applicant would handle.

6. *Clarification and reflection questions:* The interviewer may use clarification questions to reflect back the applicant's answer and thus get a fuller understanding of a question previously answered.

Employer Informational Stage

In the employer informational stage, the interviewer will attempt to obtain information about your life style, personal philosophy of life, and general character. This will involve these types of open-ended questions:

- What books have you read over the past six months?
- How have you changed over the past five years?
- As far as your work is concerned, where do you want to be in the next three years, five years, ten years?
- What hobbies do you have?
- If you could take a trip anyplace in the world, where would you go and why?

This type of open-ended question may specify a subject matter area but grant the applicant a great deal of freedom in answering. Brooks notes that, "by their nature, open-ended questions call for a response of more than a few words. Closed questions, on the other hand, place constraints upon the applicant's freedom to structure his or her own response. Closed questions call for a response of a few words."[8] Obviously, open-ended questions can elicit more information than closed questions can, but interviews that rely heavily on open-ended questions will also be far more time-consuming than those limited to closed questions.

The Windup Stage

It is important that you end the interview on a positive note, that you leave the interviewer with a positive impression of your ability, background, and personality. To accomplish this, you will have to apply in the interview the communication skills you have studied and acquired in the previous chapters.

THE DO'S AND DON'T'S OF EMPLOYMENT INTERVIEWING

Here are ten rules that nurses should keep in mind in preparing for an employment interview:

1. Do not be overly formal. Relax and be "yourself."
2. Prepare your thoughts and ideas before the interview.
3. Do not be impatient. Avoid shaking your leg, looking at your watch, or showing other signs of uneasiness.
4. Familiarize yourself with the job description and qualifications.
5. Before the interview, attempt to anticipate questions that might be asked.
6. Know something about the institution whose job you are applying for.
7. Do not be reluctant to ask questions.
8. Do not hesitate to take notes.
9. Try to establish rapport early in the interview.
10. End the interview on an appreciative note.

JOB LEADS

Table 9-3 shows the results of a survey of 6,000 newly licensed nurses conducted by the National League for Nursing and the Department of Health, Education, and Welfare.[9] The table indicates the sources of job information that nurses rate as good to excellent.

Table 9-3 Nurses' Ratings of Sources of Job Information

Sources of Information	% of Nurses
Direct application	87%
Faculty	82
Friends	76
Recruiters	73
Professional journals	68
School placement bureau	61
Nurses' conventions	59
Newspapers	54
Civil service listing	50
State nurses' association	48
State employment service	36
Commercial employment agency	35

Source: Department of Health, Education, and Welfare, 1975.

SUMMARY

It is important to remember that no two interview situations are alike. Whatever the situation, however, you should avoid putting unnecessary pressure on yourself; be open, honest, and genuine. Like politicians who prepare themselves carefully in advance of press conferences, you as a job applicant must prepare for your interview. This will help you develop a positive attitude and a self-confidence that will show that you have something positive to offer the health care community.

INTERVIEWING REVIEW PUZZLE

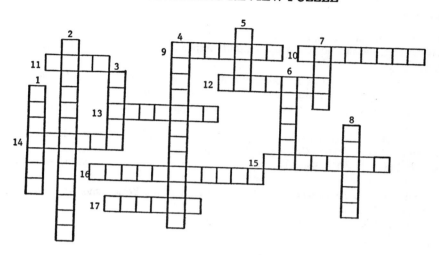

DOWN

1) Questions that are used to control the interview.
2) How should your questions be arranged?
3) Your most recent employment should be listed _____.
4) Your application letter should be _____.
5) The number of stages in a normal interview.
6) Contains vital data.
7) A type of question that is used to discover the applicant's attitude.
8) Interviewing is a _____ form of interpersonal communication.

ACROSS

9) A type of question that is used to see if the applicant is familiar with the area being examined.
10) It is important that you always be _____.
11) You can expect to speak at least _____ the time.
12) Chronological listings should be in what order?
13) You should develop this in the first stage of the interview.
14) What your answers should be.
15) You should be looking for this during the interview.
16) One of the stages in the interview process.
17) A type of question that requires few words to answer.

(Answers are on page 160.)

NOTES

1. Department of Health, Education, and Welfare, as reported in the *Nurses Almanac*, Howard S. Rowland, ed. (Germantown, Md.: Aspen Systems Corp., 1978), p. 221.
2. *Ibid*
3. Robert Goyer, Charles Redding, and John Rickey, *Interviewing Principles and Techniques* (Dubuque, Iowa: William C. Brown, 1968), p. 6.
4. William Brooks, *Speech Communication* (Dubuque, Iowa: William C. Brown, 1974), p. 194.
5. E.C. Webster, *Decision-Making in the Employment Interview* (Montreal: Industrial Relations Center, McGill University, 1964), pp. 13-14.
6. E.C. Mayfield, "The Selection Interview: A Re-evaluation of Published Research," *Personnel Psychology* 17 (1964): 239-260.
7. Arthur R. Pell, *Recruiting and Selecting Personnel* (New York: Simon and Schuster, 1969), pp. 105-106.
8. Brooks, *Speech Communication*, pp. 196-197.
9. DHEW, p. 217.

SUGGESTED READINGS

Amsden, Forrest M., and White, Noel D. *How To Be Successful in the Employment Interview: A Step-by-Step Approach for the Candidate*. Cheney, Wash.: Interviewing Dynamics, 1975.

Basset, Glenn A. *Practical Interviewing: A Handbook for Managers*. New York: American Management Association, 1965.

Bingham, W., Moore, B., and Gustad, J. *How To Interview*. New York: Harper & Row, 1959.

Cannell, C.F., Fisher, G., and Baker, T. "Reporting of Hospitalization in the Health Interview Survey: A Methodological Study of Several Factors Affecting the Reporting of Hospital Episodes." *Health Statistics from the National Health Survey*. Washington, D.C.: Public Health Service, Publication No. 584-D4, May, 1961.

――――, and Kahn, R.L. "Interviewing." In *The Handbook of Social Psychology*, edited by G. Lindzey and E. Aronson. Reading, Mass.: Addison Wesley, 1968, pp. 526-595.

Carlson, R.E., Schwab, D.P., and Henneman, H.G. "Agreement Among Selection Interview Styles." *Journal of Industrial Psychology* 5: 8-17.

Goyer, Robert S., Redding, Charles W., and Rickey, John T. *Interviewing Principles and Techniques: A Project Text*. Dubuque, Iowa: William C. Brown, 1968.

Kahn, Robert L., and Cannell, Charles F. *The Dynamics of Interviewing*. New York: John Wiley and Sons, Inc., 1964.

Kindall, A., and Gatza, J. "Positive Program of Performance Appraisal." *Harvard Business Review* 41: 153-160.

Lahiff, J. "Interviewing for Results." In *Readings in Interpersonal and Organizational Communication*, edited by R. Huseman, C. Logue, and D. Freshley. Boston: Holbrook Press, 1975, pp. 332-353.

Mayfield, E. "The Selection Interview: A Reevaluation of Published Research." *Personnel Psychology* 17: 239-260.

Pell, Arthur R. *Recruiting and Selecting Personnel.* New York: Simon and Schuster, 1969.

Shouksmith, G. *Assessment Through Interviewing.* London: Pergamon, 1968.

Steward, C., and Cash, W. *Interviewing: Principles and Practices.* Dubuque, Iowa: William C. Brown, 1974.

Webster, E.C. *Decision-Making in the Employment Interview.* Montreal: Industrial Relations Center, McGill University, 1964.

Wright, O. "Summary of Research on the Selection Interview Since 1964." *Personnel Psychology* 22: 391-413.

Zima, Joseph. "Interviewing: An Imperative Interpersonal Communication Skill." In *Explorations in Speech Communication,* edited by John McKay. Columbus, Ohio: Merrill Publishing, 1973, pp. 91-107.

INTERVIEWING REVIEW PUZZLE

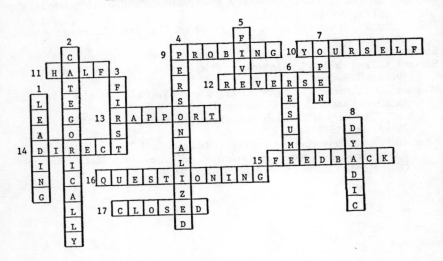

DOWN

1) Questions that are used to control the interview.
2) How should your questions be arranged?
3) Your most recent employment should be listed _____.
4) Your application letter should be _____.
5) The number of stages in a normal interview.
6) Contains vital data.
7) A type of question that is used to discover the applicant's attitude.
8) Interviewing is a _____ form of interpersonal communication.

ACROSS

9) A type of question that is used to see if the applicant is familiar with the area being examined.
10) It is important that you always be _____.
11) You can expect to speak at least _____ the time.
12) Chronological listings should be in what order?
13) You should develop this in the first stage of the interview.
14) What your answers should be.
15) You should be looking for this during the interview.
16) One of the stages in the interview process.
17) A type of question that requires few words to answer.

Appendix A

Programmed Chapter Review

This appendix contains a programmed chapter review of the material covered in the book. The answers are in the column to the left of the questions. Cover the answers with a note card and lower the card after you answer each question. If you give an incorrect response, go back and review the appropriate chapter before continuing with the review:

CHAPTER 1

Abraham Maslow

Maslow

hierarchy

perceives

communication

empathic

ask, persuade
tell, demand

sensitive

private

openly

maximum

1. The early work of _____ still serves as the main source of motivational theory today.
_____ contended that we are motivated by a _____ of human needs.
2. Communication between a supervisor and subordinate will result in what the subordinate _____ it to be.
3. The better supervisors tend to be _____ minded.
4. The better supervisors tend to be _____ listeners.
5. The better supervisors tend to _____ or _____ rather than _____ or _____.
6. The better supervisors tend to be _____ to the feelings and ego-defense needs of their subordinates. They are careful to reprimand in _____ rather than in public.
7. The better supervisors _____ pass along information.
8. High job satisfaction and quality patient care depend upon the _____ use of the individual's training and skill.

correlation

participation

mutually
build

lacking
absent
money
security

money
long-

fifth
interesting work

direct

decreases

setting
congruent

common

false

not

9. There is a positive _____ between performance and one's job attitude and the degree of _____ in the decision-making process.

10. Herzberg, like Maslow, found that motivational needs are not _____ exclusive but rather that one may _____ on another.

11. Remember that maintenance factors created job dissatisfaction only when they were _____ or _____ from the job.

12. It takes more than just _____ and _____ to motivate nurses.

13. Most motivational theorists will tell you that _____ is not a _____lasting motivator.

14. The Michigan Survey Research Center discovered that good pay came in _____ behind _____.

15. When nurses become less involved in _____ patient care their job satisfaction level _____.

16. Consequently, the nurse becomes dissatisfied with the practice _____.

17. Only through _____ perceptions can we solve problems and work together toward a _____ goal.

18. Too many times our perceptions of another's needs are _____ perceptions.

19. What motivates you might _____ motivate someone else.

belongingness

20. Most motivational theorists believe that most employees are motivated by managers who stress the _____ and esteem needs of their employees.

bottom
top

21. Japanese business organizations believe that the most important information flows from the _____ up and not from the _____ down.

humanistic
relations
production

22. The organizational climate in Japan is centered around _____ psychology in which human _____ are just as important as _____.

CHAPTER 2

perception

23. Organizational climate is a multidimensional _____ of the organization by its members.

behavioral

24. Perceptions, whether real or unreal, have _____ consequences for the organization.

similar, different

25. Organizational climate is both _____ to and _____ from the weather.

see, touch
sense

26. Unlike weather, the organizational climate in a hospital is not something that we can directly _____ or _____, but we can _____ it.

environment
change

27. People create their own work _____; therefore, if it's not right, people can _____ it.

high

28. Numerous studies have shown that certain types of organizational climate typify _____ performance groups.

behavior

balance

six
two

cohesion

aspiration

influence

influenced

comparison
trust
performance

supportive

own

affect, relationships

conditions

morale

collective

29. The _____ nurses exhibit on the job helps to determine organizational climate.
30. Highly cohesive groups have more communicative _____ than groups of low cohesion.
31. There are _____ climate dimensions divided into _____ groups.
32. The greater the group's _____, the more power it has to bring about conformity to its norms.
33. A group's _____ level helps determine its degree of success or failure.
34. Members of cohesive groups more readily exert _____ over one another and are more readily _____ by one another than are members of low cohesive groups.
35. When joining a group, a person employs a standard called the _____ level.
36. High _____ tends to stimulate high _____ and increases employee confidence, loyalty, and teamwork.
37. Highly motivated individuals tend to work in _____ organizational climates.
38. We live in climates of our _____ making and these self made climates _____ our _____ with others.
39. The working _____ and employees' perceptions of those conditions affect individual _____ and determine the climate in which they work.
40. Organizational climate is the _____ view of the people

environment

CHAPTER 3

practice

efficiency

data
grievances
special

hear
analyze, recall
conclusions

understand

45
talking
16
writing

half

receiving
sending

Feedback, certified

four

within an organization as to the nature of the _____ in which they work.

41. Listening proficiency can be improved with _____.
42. Listening can mean greater _____.
43. Listening is needed to gather necessary _____.
44. Listening helps in settling ____.
45. Listening makes people feel ____.
46. Deliberative listening is the ability to _____ information, to _____ it, to _____ it at a later time, and to draw _____ from it.
47. In deliberative listening, one strives to _____ the message.
48. Research shows that average working adults divide their communication time roughly along these lines: reading, _____ percent; _____, 30 percent; reading, _____ percent and _____, 9 percent.
49. These statistics indicate that almost _____ of your communication time is spent in listening.
50. If you defined communication with emphasis on the _____ end as well as on the _____ end, you recognized the importance of listening.
51. _____ is the _____ mail of listening.
52. There are _____ types of listening responses.

like

positive

up, down
Attention, interest

nonverbal
two

delivery

ideas
feelings

bias

fake

interrupt

frame of reference
500

125

one-third
one-half
eight

53. One kind of behavior normally brings about a _____ behavior.
54. People tend to do things well when they hold _____ labels about their ability to do them.
55. There is a human tendency to live _____ or _____ to labels.
56. _____ and _____ are synonymous.
57. You should learn to watch for the speaker's verbal as well as _____ messages.
58. Everyone sends ____ messages.
59. You should not decide from the appearance or _____ of speakers that what they have to say is worthwhile.
60. You should listen for _____ and underlying _____.
61. You should try to determine your own _____, if any, and try to allow for it.
62. Too many times we _____ attention to the speaker.
63. You should not _____ immediately if you hear a statement that you feel is wrong.
64. You should try to see the situation from the other person's _____.
65. Our minds function at _____ words per minute, but we normally speak at _____ words per minute.
66. Studies at Florida State and Michigan State Universities showed that people forget ____ to _____ of what they hear within _____ hours.

CHAPTER 4

intense

ears
all

feedback

stress

four

judge

suspend

feelings

attending, responding

physical

38
55, facial
four

swap

verify

parasupporting
Cliches

67. To be a good listener requires
_____ concentration.
68. We do not listen only with our
_____.
69. We should listen for _____
meanings.
70. To be effective, the nurse must
listen for _____.
71. Listening can reduce unnecessary patient _____.
72. The good listener must meet
_____ prerequisites before enter-
ing into a helping relationship.
73. The major barrier to interpersonal communication is our very
natural tendency to _____.
74. The listener must be willing to
_____ judgment.
75. The listener must allow and encourage the statement of _____
by the sender.
76. The listener promotes empathy
by _____ and _____
responses.
77. The nonverbal cues that indicate
the listener is attending are primarily _____.
78. Of the total message, 7 percent
is verbal, _____ percent is vocal,
and _____ percent is _____.
79. There are _____ rules of
paraphrasing.
80. Don't just word _____.
81. Give the other person a chance
to _____ your paraphrase.
82. The second dimension of perception checking is called _____.
83. _____ put distance between
communicators.
84. A mere repetition of what the

empathy

CHAPTER 5

social

group dynamics

two
task, individual

done

people

exclusive

task
individual

task

individual

competent

behaves

tension
satisfy
arbitrary

other has said does little to
establish _____.

85. From the _____ sciences
emerged the concept of
_____ with its focus
upon members of the group
rather than solely on the leader.
86. The _____ main components of
leadership are _____ and _____
behavior.
87. The task-oriented leader is
mainly interested in getting the
job _____.
88. The individually oriented leader
is mainly interested in _____.
89. However, the task and individual functions of leadership are
not mutually _____.
90. Group member satisfaction is
high when a leader emerges who
is effective both in _____ and
_____ group functions, or two
complementary leaders emerge
and one handles the _____ functions of the group while the
other handles the _____ functions, and when the designated
leader or leaders are perceived to
be _____ by the group
members.
91. Members of a group might begin
to behave toward others in much
the same way their leader
_____ toward them.
92. Persuasive climates reduced
_____ and tended to
_____ personal needs more
than _____ climates.

forget

93. Effective leaders often _____ about a problem for a while in order to solve it.

94. Leadership effectiveness is dependent upon the _____.

situation

different

95. Leaders cannot be too _____ from their followers.

identify

96. Followers must be able to _____ with their leader.

97. Early studies on leadership depended almost exclusively on the _____ approach.

trait

trait

static

98. The _____ approach examined only the _____ characteristics of people; it did not describe the dynamics of leadership as a

process

_____.

99. Behavior by an undesignated leader is often referred to as the _____ of _____ leadership.

dynamics, personal

four

100. The leader can exhibit only ____ possible leadership behaviors. These behaviors are:

High, high

101. _____ task and _____ individual behavior.

task, individual

102. High _____ and low _____ behavior.

low

103. High individual and _____ task behavior.

Low, low

104. _____ task and _____ individual behavior.

high

high

environmental

training

development

105. A nurse's degree of job satisfaction is highest when the leadership exhibits _____ task and _____ individual behavior.

106. Research indicates that _____ factors and proper _____ play a significant role in the _____ of leadership abilities.

directive

autocratic

107. Automatic and habitual reactions portray highly _____, _____ leadership.

work, interact

followers
followers
leader

attitudes
followers

CHAPTER 6

nonverbal

language

congruent

meaningful

dependent

silence

communicate
not

credibility

six

clear
verbal

108. Research has shown that leaders should be selected on the basis of how they _____ and _____ with the people they are to lead.
109. A leader must have _____, for without _____ there is no need for a _____.
110. The behavior of leaders will be determined to a large extent by the _____ and training of their _____.

111. The real distinction between verbal and _____ communication is that verbal communication is organized by a _____ system.
112. When the nonverbal message is _____ and tends to support the verbal message, we have clear, _____ communication.
113. Body language and spoken language are _____ upon each other.
114. In its proper context, even _____ is communication.
115. Patients may choose to stop talking but they do not cease to _____.
116. We cannot choose _____ to communicate.
117. Nonverbal behaviors normally have a high degree of _____ in the mind of the beholder.
118. There are _____ basic facial expressions.
119. Most nonverbal theorists agree that if the meaning of the facial expression is _____ but the _____ context in which it

face

personalized

like
dislike

eye contact

tension

tone

verbal
attitudes

space

spatial

Distance, space

bubble

three

Intimate

5

5, 100

occurs is not, then the _____
is the most reliable source.

120. Eye contact is a highly _____
form of nonverbal communication.

121. We tend to look at things we
_____ and to look away from
things we _____.

122. When two people like one
another, they establish _____
more often and for longer dura-
tions than when there is _____
in the relationship.

123. The _____ of the voice conveys different meanings.

124. Research indicates that touch
behavior by nurses increases
_____ output by patients and
improves the patients' _____
toward the nurses.

125. We all carry our personal _____
and status around with us as we
stake out our territory within
the limits of our influence.

126. Individuals send messages by
placing themselves in certain
_____ relationships with one
another.

127. _____ and _____ tell nurses
things about their working relationships.

128. Personal space can be thought of
as a plastic _____ that surrounds the individual.

129. There are _____ major interpersonal distances. These are:

130. _____ distance, 3 to 20
inches.

131. Social distance, 20 inches to _____
feet.

132. Public distance, _____ feet to _____
feet.

social

133. Nonverbal behavior must be interpreted in its proper _____ context.

CHAPTER 7

collection

134. A group is a _____ of individuals.

Delete

135. _____ one member from a group and that group changes in character.

people

136. The characteristics of a group are determined by the _____ comprising the group.

information, knowledge

137. Learning groups attempt to impart new _____ or _____ to all group members.

task

138. Policy-making groups are usually _____ centered.

should
implement, policy
High-
low-

139. The role of a decision-making group is not to consider what _____ be policy but how to _____ established _____.

140. _____status members tend to communicate more than _____ status members.

High-

141. _____status members tend to communicate more with other _____status members.

high-
Low-
high-

142. _____status members tend to communicate more with _____ status members than with other _____status members.

low-

talking

143. There is a high correlation between the rank of group members and the amount of _____ they do within their group.

shared

144. A group norm is the _____ acceptance of a rule.

difficult

145. The longer a group member waits to speak, the more _____ it becomes.

cohesive

five

five
cohesion

satisfaction

small, large
circular
seen

dominant

four
wheel
chain, all-channel

all-channel

defensiveness

spontaneity

permissiveness

skills
interests

status, all

group

146. Social pressure is highest in groups that are highly _____.

147. The ideal size for small group efficiency is _____ members.

148. Most authorities tend to agree that, as group size increases beyond _____ members, there is less group _____.

149. Members of five-man groups express complete _____; they do not regard their groups either as too _____ or as too _____.

150. Sitting in a _____ pattern, in which everyone can be _____ and no one is in a physically _____ position, may help to create a more open and friendly atmosphere.

151. There are _____ main communication networks: _____, _____, circle, and _____.

152. Most authorities seem to agree that, in most cases, the _____ is the most suitable.

153. The simplest spoken question, even when it comes from a professional, may evoke _____.

154. Nurses in staff meetings should look for _____ rather than manipulation.

155. Effective groups tend to have a high degree of _____.

156. Effective groups assign tasks on the basis of people's _____ and _____.

157. Effective groups exhibit intragroup _____ where _____ members share in the recognition and rewards of _____ achievement.

158. Just because someone disagrees with us does not necessarily

dislike

disagreement
personal
mutual

CHAPTER 8

misinterpretation

Meaning
words

Semantics

symbol

referent

symbols, signs

symbols

animals

shortcuts

2,000

14

verbal, situational

code

mean they _____ us.
159. It is essential to discriminate accurately between _____ and _____ dislike if we are going to solve _____ problems cooperatively.

160. Poor communication is the result of _____ and misunderstanding.
161. _____ is in the person.
162. We assume _____ have meaning.
163. _____ is the study of words; it is concerned with the relationship between a _____ and the thing it represents, called a _____.
164. We use both _____ and _____ to communicate.
165. The use of _____ is one of the basic characteristics that separates humans from _____.
166. In a way, symbols are communication _____.
167. The number of words an adult uses in daily conversation is about _____.
168. The 500 words used the most in the English language have at least ____ thousand different definitions.
169. The nurse must be able to discriminate accurately between the _____ and _____ contexts of messages.
170. We can communicate clearly only if we are using the same communicative _____.

What
meaning
word-
person-
paraphrase

distorted

CHAPTER 9

first

interstate

Nonfinancial
financial

dyadic

checklist

employment

specialty

state, nursing

openings

personalized

171. You should never ask, "Do you understand?" Ask instead, "_____ do you understand?"
172. Words have no _____.
173. Do not be _____minded.
174. Be _____minded.
175. Question and _____ what has been said.
176. When messages are passed from one person to another, there is a tendency for the message to become _____.

177. The employment moves of nurses usually occur within the _____ few years of graduation from nursing school.
178. Nurses are almost as willing to make _____ as intrastate moves.
179. _____ incentives appear to appeal more than _____ incentives to the single R.N. who is considering a move.
180. Interviewing is a _____ form of interpersonal communication.
181. A _____ of your interests and qualifications is the essential first step to take before the _____ interview.
182. It is usually best to apply only to hospitals with openings in your _____.
183. For out-of-state jobs, contact the _____ board of _____.
184. Compare your initial checklist with available hospital _____.
185. Your application letter should be _____.
186. The original covering letter should be neatly and freshly

bond
8½-by-11

business
resume

reverse

welcome

categories
eye

words

nonrepetitive
honest

rapport

four, five

half
"W"

Leading

Probing

typed on white _____ paper,
_____ inches.

187. The application letter should be in proper _____ form.
188. The _____ contains vital data about your education, experience, and skills.
189. Chronological listings of education and experience should be in _____ order.
190. Most interviewers not only expect but _____ questions from you during the interview.
191. It is usually best to group your questions into _____.
192. Maintain _____ contact with the interviewer.
193. The interviewer and applicant cannot depend upon _____ alone.
194. Be direct in your answers, _____ in your questions, and _____ in the discussion of your goals.
195. It is essential that you quickly establish _____ with the interviewer.
196. Interviewers tend to form initial impressions about applicants within the first ____ or ____ minutes of the interview.
197. You can expect to talk at least _____ of the time.
198. ____ questions are used in most interviewing situations.
199. _____ questions may be used to control the interview.
200. _____ questions are used to discover the applicant's familiarity with the area being examined.

Index

questioning, 153, 154
warmup, 153
windup, 155

J

Job. *See* Employment

K

Kelly, H.H., 28, 29
Kelley, Charles, 39, 53

L

Leaders
  activities, 80
  behavior, 68
  feeling in, 6, 7
  groups, 69
    norms, 108
    status, 107
  nurses, 67, 68
  orientation, 68, 69
  selection
    interactional approach, 70–73
    trait approach, 69, 70
  style questionnaire, 73–79
  teamwork, 29
  See also Nursing Supervisors
Leads
  employment, 155, 156
Learning Groups. *See* Groups
Leavitt, Harold, 111
Letter. *See* Application Letter
Lewin, Kurt, 67
License
  resume, 150
Likert, Renis, 29
Listening
  active, 53
    importance, 54, 55
    improvement, 59, 60

skills, 56–59
  activities, 48–50
  deliberative, 39
    improvement, 59, 60
  evaluation, 45
  feigning interest, 44, 45
  health care professionals,
    40, 41, 46
  patient care, 37
  proficiency, 39
  reflection, 45
  responses, 41, 42
  skills, 42–45
  time and effort, 39, 40
  verbal vs. nonverbal messages,
    44
Listening Skills. *See* Listening

M

McGregor, Douglas, 4
Maintenance Factors
  job dissatisfaction, 7
Maslow, Abraham, 4
Mayfield, E.C., 153
Mehrabian, Albert, 57, 88, 91
Miller, N.E., 68
Meaning
  fallacy, 128
  people, 130
Messages
  activities, 139
  context, 131, 132
  deliberative listening, 39
  distortion, 134, 135
  nonverbal
    impact, 88
    vs. verbal, 44, 45
Metzger, Norman, 59, 60
Michigan State University.
  See Universities
Minnesota Mining and
  Manufacturing, 39
Mobility
  nurse, 147, 148

North Carolina State University,
87
Ohio State, 70
University of Florida, 45
University of Michigan, 10
University of Minnesota, 45

V

Verbosity
dysfunctional response, 59

W

Wages
employment interview, 152
needs, 10
Warmup Stage
employment interview, 153

Weaver, Richard, 53, 54
Webster, E.C., 88
Western Electric, 39
Wheel
communication network, 111
White, A.G., 92
Windup Stage
interview, 155
Words
meaning, 130, 131
technical use, 132–134
Work
appreciation, 5
challenging, 8, 9
See also Employment

Z

Zander, Alvin, 27, 106

About the Author

Harry E. Munn, Jr., is an Associate Professor of Organizational Communication at North Carolina State University in Raleigh. He received his Bachelor of Science degree from the University of Wisconsin and his Master of Arts degree from Bradley University in Speech Communication. His Ph.D. is from the University of Kansas in Speech Communication and Human Relations.

Prior to teaching at North Carolina State he taught at Kent State University, the University of Florida, and the University of Kansas.

He has written extensively in health care journals and is on the editorial board of *Hospital Topics*. He is, as well, a consultant to a wide range of national and regional health care organizations. He has spoken to, and participated in seminars for nursing groups, hospitals, clinics, and health care associations from coast to coast.